First published in Great Britain in 2013 by

Policy Press
University of Bristol
Fourth Floor
Beacon House
Queen's Road
Bristol BS8 1QU
UK
t:+44 (0)117 331 4054
f: +44 (0)117 331 4093
tpp-info@bristol.ac.uk
www.policypress.co.uk

North America office:
Policy Press
c/o The University of Chicago Press
1427 East 60th Street
Chicago, IL 60637, USA
t: +1 773 702 7700
f: +1 773-702-9756
sales@press.uchicago.edu
www.press.uchicago.edu

British Library Cataloguing in Publication Data
A catalogue record for this book is available from the British Library.

Library of Congress Cataloging-in-Publication Data
A catalog record for this book has been requested.

ISBN 978 1 44730 637 5 hardcover

Cover design by www.thecoverfactory.co.uk
Front cover: image kindly supplied by istock
Printed and bound in Great Britain by TJ International, Padstow
Policy Press uses environmentally responsible print partners.

MIX
Paper from responsible sources
FSC® C013056
www.fsc.org

ORGANISING WASTE IN THE CITY

International perspectives on narratives and practices

Edited by
María José Zapata Campos
and C. Michael Hall

Contents

Part IV: Waste and environmental, economic and social justice

List of figures and tables

Figures

Tables

Abbreviations

AECID	Spanish Agency for International Development Cooperation
ANCI	Associazione Nazionale Comuni Italiani (National Association of the Italian Municipalities), Italy
ANT	actor-network theory
APE	Association for the Protection of the Environment, Egypt
ARO	ambito di raccolta ottimale (optimal collection area), Italy
ARPA	Agenzia Regionale per la Prevenzione e la Protezione Ambientale (Regional Agency for Environmental Prevention and Protection), Italy
ASM	Azienda Servizi Municipalizzati (municipal urban waste company), Molfetta, Italy
ATO	ambito territoriale ottimale (optimal territorial area), Italy
AVR	Afvalverwerking Rijnmond (Waste Management Service Rijnmond), the Netherlands
CCBA	Cairo Cleaning and Beautification Authority, Egypt
CID	Community and Institutional Development
CLG	Department for Communities and Local Government, UK
CO_2	carbon dioxide
CoNaI	Consorzio Nazionale Imballaggi (National Packaging Consortium), Italy
CoReVe	Consorzio Recupero Vetro (Italian Glass Recycle Consortium), Italy
CRV	Centro Raccolta Vetro (Recycling Glass Centre), Trani, Italy
CURE	Centrum Uitvoering Reinigingstaken Eindhoven en omgeving (Centre for Waste Management Tasks Eindhoven and surroundings), the Netherlands
DEFRA	Department for Environment, Food and Rural Affairs, UK
DETR	Department of the Environment, Transport and the Regions, UK
DoE	Department of the Environment, UK
DoH	Department of Health, UK
DTI	Department for Trade and Industry, UK
EEAA	Egyptian Environmental Affairs Agency

EPC	Environmental Protection Company, Egypt
EQI	Environmental Quality International
ERSAP	Economic Reform and Structural Adjustment Programme, EU
ESRC	Economic and Social Research Council, UK
EU	European Union
FAO	Food and Agriculture Organisation of the United Nations
FoE	Friends of the Earth
HMS	Haagse Milieu Services (The Hague Environmental Services), the Netherlands
IES	International Environment Services
IFI	international financial institutions
IMF	International Monetary Fund
INCPEN	Industrial Council for Packaging and the Environment
IPC	Integrated Pollution Control
ISPRA	Istituto Superiore per la Protezione e la Ricerca Ambientale (Institute for Environmental Protection and Research), Italy
ISWH	International Sustainable Waste Hierarchy
ISWM	Integrated Solid Waste Management
LEG	Lockleaze Environment Group
LEGFG	Lockleaze Environment Group Focus Group
MP	Member of Parliament
NGO	non-governmental organisation
NIMBY	not in my backyard
NSR	Nordvästra Skånes Renhållnings AB (Northwest Scania Recycling Ltd), Sweden
ODPM	Office of the Deputy Prime Minister, UK
OECD	Organisation for Economic Co-operation and Development
ONS	Office for National Statistics, UK
PPP	public–private partnership
RMA	Resource Management Act, New Zealand
SDRN	Sustainable Development Research Network
TDs	Teachta Dàla, or public representatives and members of the Dáil
UN-Habitat	United Nations Human Settlements Programme
UNDP	United Nations Development Programme
UNECE	United Nations Economic Commission for Europe
WMMP	Waste Management and Minimisation Plans
ZEDP	Zabaleen Environmental Development Programme

Notes on contributors

Karen Bell is a research associate in the Centre for the Study of Poverty and Social Justice, at University of Bristol, UK. Her current research and interests include environmental justice; the political economy of sustainability; degrowth in relation to poverty reduction; community empowerment; and class, 'race' and disability equality. Karen was formerly a community development worker in Bristol.

Hervé Corvellec is professor of business administration at the Department of Service Management, Lund University, Sweden. He has a distinct theoretical interest for narratives, argumentation and rhetoric, and a research focus on infrastructures such as waste management, public transportation, energy provision and cultural institutions.

Anna Davies is professor of geography at Trinity College Dublin, Ireland, where she directs the Environmental Governance Research Group. In addition to extensive work on waste, Anna's research interests in the area of environmental governance also include sustainable consumption and enterprise, climate change and biodiversity. Recent publications on waste include *Garbage governance* (Ashgate, 2008), *Enterprising communities* (Emerald, 2012) and 'The geography and the matter of waste mobilities' (*Transactions of the Institute of British Geographers*, 2012).

Wael Fahmi was trained as an architect at Cairo University, Egypt, and received his PhD in planning and landscape from the University of Manchester, UK. He teaches architecture design and urban conservation of historical districts as professor at the Architecture Department, Helwan University, Cairo. Wael and Keith Sutton have published two books on New Cairo's *Fragmented city* and on the *Rehabilitation of Cairo's historical districts*; a book on Cairo's planning and housing issues is forthcoming.

C. Michael Hall is professor at the Department of Management, University of Canterbury, New Zealand; he is also docent at the Department of Geography, University of Oulu, Finland; visiting professor, Centre for Tourism Studies, University of Eastern Finland, Savolinna and Linnaeus University School of Business and Economics, Linnaeus University, Kalmar, Sweden; and fellow at Freiburg Institute of Advanced Studies, Germany. He is the author of numerous works in the areas of environmental change, heritage, regional development, sustainable consumption, food and tourism.

Johan Hultman is professor in human geography at the Department of Service Management, Lund University, Sweden. He has developed theoretical interests in the intersections between mobility, nature and materialities, and entertains a bi-focal research interest on waste and tourism.

Philip Marcel Karré is programme director and lecturer in urban management and public administration at the Amsterdam University of Applied Sciences. He wrote his PhD thesis on hybrid organisations in waste management (see www.hybridorganizations.com).

Liam Leonard is college lecturer in environmentalism, criminology, sociology and human rights at the Institute of Technology, Sligo, Ireland. He is the author of over 10 books, including a study on the Irish and Greek 'crisis of the peripheries' and an analysis of the environmental movement in Ireland. He is chair of the Criminology Association of Ireland and formerly president of the Sociology Association of Ireland. In addition, he edited the 2010 special issue of the *Environmental Politics Journal* and was guest editor for the civil society issue of the *Irish Journal of Sociology*.

Dario Minervini has a PhD in sociology and social research and is currently research fellow at the Department of Social Sciences, University of Naples 'Federico II', Italy. His teaching activities concern the area of environmental sociology. He is involved in several research projects relating to sociotechnical innovation, environmental governance as well as emerging green jobs. He is the author of *Politica e rifiuti* [*Politics and waste*] (Liguori, 2010). His research interests concern the multilevel waste policies and processes of professionalisation in the field of the green economy.

Keith Sutton graduated from University College London researching into the historical geography of France. Prior to retiring he was senior lecturer in geography at the University of Manchester, UK. He has published numerous articles and chapters on aspects of economic and social development and on rural settlement in Algeria and on rural development in Malaysia. More recently he has focused on urban planning and heritage issues in Cairo.

David Sweeting is senior lecturer in urban studies in the School of Policy Studies at the University of Bristol, UK. He developed an interest in issues pertaining to waste and recycling through research into local government strategies in this area. He teaches on environmental issues at undergraduate and postgraduate levels.

María José Zapata Campos has a PhD in sociology. She is a research fellow in the Managing Big Cities programme at the Gothenburg Research Institute, University of Gothenburg, Sweden. She is also engaged in the research programme 'Organising critical infrastructure services – A case study of waste management' led by the Service Management Department, Lund University, Sweden. Her current research deals with city management and issues of sustainability in cities, the sociology of organisations, tourism and development studies.

Patrik Zapata, PhD, is associate professor at the School of Public Administration, University of Gothenburg, Sweden. His research deals with the management of cities, sustainable organising, scandalology, language in organisations and relations between organisations.

Acknowledgements

This book draws together contributions from an international group of scholars committed to undertaking research about the many faces of waste from a critical social sciences perspective. Their previous research has been an inspiration to us to edit a book about how waste is being organised in cities, and the implications of this for sustainable development.

The origins of this book lay with a conversation with David Sweeting. We had recently started reading, lecturing and doing research about waste, and were equally fascinated about the many sociopolitical dimensions of this issue, and how they were as yet uncovered by the existing literature. It is fair to say that, without David's first conversations with the publishers and his input into the book proposal, this book would not have appeared.

The book also benefited from a seminar held in Gothenburg, Sweden, in September 2011, where the book's contributors met to discuss their preliminary chapters. The richness of the discussions was invaluable.

Despite the individual funding behind each, the book would not have been possible without the research institutions that sponsored our work. We therefore acknowledge the support from the research projects: 'Organising sustainability in the glocalised city', funded by the Jan Wallander Foundation, Sweden; 'Waste in translation. How ideas of waste management travel from global to local', funded by the Gothenburg Centre of Globalization and Development, University of Gothenburg; and 'Organising critical infrastructure services – A case study of waste management', funded by the Swedish Governmental Agency for Innovation Systems (VINNOVA). Michael would also like to acknowledge the support of the Freiburg Institute for Advanced Studies for a space – complete with urban wasteland – in which to be able to complete the book, as well as Jody, Cooper and JC for the conversion of his own wasteland.

Finally, we wish to acknowledge the people that take away our waste, the drivers of the waste trucks, the informal scavengers in Gothenburg, the waste pickers in La Chureca rubbish dump, the Zabaleen and their 'Garbage City', and the ordinary citizens who daily commit to reduce their waste and dare to look into their rubbish.

ONE

Introduction: narratives of organising waste in the city

María José Zapata Campos and C. Michael Hall

The challenges of climate and environmental change and the contribution of cities to global warming and natural resource depletion make the issue of sustainable urban waste governance crucial for contemporary urban spaces and for their wider ecological footprint. However, while some of the issues surrounding the governance of waste have been identified in the contemporary literature, relatively little attention has been given to the various, often highly contested, ways in which waste and its governance are framed. This book offers a critical social sciences perspective on the issue of organising waste in cities. Often positioned in terms of relatively narrow engineering, economic and/or physical scientific discourses (see, for example, Barton et al, 1996; Morrissey and Browne, 2004; Skordilis, 2004; Hung et al, 2007), the book aims to emphasise the ways in which the notion of waste, and the narratives and discourses associated with it, are socially constructed with corresponding implications for the governance of waste and local waste handling practices (see, for example, Cooper, 2009; Tuler and Webler, 2010; Fried and Eyles, 2011; Corvellec and Hultman, 2012; Foote and Mazzolini, 2012). Therefore, the contributions contained in this book position the governance of waste not from a specific managerial perspective but from a range of different understandings of how the waste problem is defined, interpreted and governed. The focus of the book is on urban and municipal household solid waste, but concerns over waste are linked to such issues as globalisation, governance, biodiversity and social, economic and environmental justice.

The popular saying, 'Your rubbish is someone else's treasure,' is not just an indication of the marketisation of waste, but also the way in which waste is socially constructed (see, for example, Douglas, 1966; MacKillop, 2009). The meanings of waste, and therefore the values attached to it, varies between places, societies, cultures, economies, markets, spaces and times. The waste infrastructures created to store waste become a mirror, making it possible to understand how society resembles it by providing its reflection (see Chapter Three, this volume).

In other words, waste becomes a narrative/narrator of the society in which it is embedded. However, waste is much more than a social construct: 'Waste is intrinsically, profoundly, a matter of materiality' (Gregson and Crang, 2010: 1026). The concept of the 'sociomateriality' of waste referred to in some chapters of this book (see Chapters Five and Eight, for example) relates to the way we engage with the materiality of waste in the course of our everyday lives (Gregson, 2009; Corvellec and Hultman, 2012; Hultman and Corvellec, 2012), as producers of waste, as politicians, as waste managers, as citizens, or as waste collectors (see also Hawkins, 2006, 2009, 2010; Lane and Gorman-Murray, 2011). For many urban residents, for example, waste recycling bins take new space in our kitchen, its odour remains in our homes after our bins have been emptied, and we are increasingly exhorted to look into our waste to sort it out, classify it, clean it and dispose of it (Bulkeley and Gregson, 2009) before, in much of the global North at least, it enters the 'black box' (Latour, 1987) of the waste management and recycling process, away from the eyes and nose of much of the urban population. To examine such narratives the book draws together contributions from an international group of scholars undertaking research in this field from a multiplicity of disciplines within the social sciences: the sociology of environment and technology, social policy, public administration, political science, management and organisation studies, urban studies, geography and urban ecology.

Social life is a narrative (MacIntyre, 1981), and narratives in social sciences research are usually understood as 'a spoken or written text giving an account of an event/action or series of events/actions, chronologically connected' (Czarniawska, 2004: 17). Having also considered the relevant social dimension of waste and its sociomateriality, it is not by chance that a book about waste from the social sciences perspective is a book about narratives. However, the chapters in the book use narratives in different ways. Some specifically address global narratives of waste as the object of their analysis. This is the case of the zero waste movement (see Chapters Four and Ten), the International Sustainable Waste Hierarchy (ISWH) (see Chapters Four and Five), or the European waste hierarchy model (Hultman and Corvellec, 2012; see also Chapter Eight). As societal narratives, these narratives of waste 'reflect and affect the specificities of the societies where they emerge' (Corvellec and Hultman, 2012: 298). Hall (Chapter Two) also introduces his chapter with a discussion of Christian narratives of wasteland, and how this transformed the way that concepts of nature and the place of nature in Western society have been constructed. Other chapters deal with narratives and constructions of waste as a method to inquire data: in Chapter Five, Zapata is inspired by deconstruction methods (Martin, 1990) to understand how global narratives of waste produced by UN-Habitat are locally translated. Finally, other chapters collect individual, personal or local narratives of waste. Accordingly, Fahmi and Sutton (Chapter Nine) collect narratives of rubbish collectors to examine the impacts of waste policies privatisation at Cairo; Bell and Sweeting (Chapter Eleven) collect stories about waste recycling in the neighbourhood where they live in Bristol; Minervini (Chapter Six) shadows his own wine bottle and narrates its journey until it becomes part of the glass purchased by a multinational corporation in Italy; and Zapata Campos (Chapter Three) uses narratives of waste from the cities of Managua in Nicaragua and Gothenburg in Sweden to rethink the functions of waste urban infrastructures.

The book takes a broad and international approach to the ways in which the issue of waste in cities is framed, with insights from within and beyond Europe. It brings together narratives of how contemporary cities around the world deal with the governance of its waste. Disparate cities such as Amsterdam, Bristol, Cairo, Gothenburg, Helsingborg and Managua are brought together. In this book cities are understood as ordinary rather than Western, 'third world', developed or global (Robinson, 2006: 1), as they are normally labelled. Instead, by focusing on ordinary cities, global and local divisions and geographies are transcended and we succeed in learning from all the experiences through comparison (Scheinberg et al, 2010).

The chapters have been organised into four sections that disclose the aim of this book: spaces, places and sites of waste in the city; global waste discourses and narratives shaping local practices; waste governance and management practices; and how civil society is responding and sometimes contesting waste policies, and what issues of environmental, economic and social injustice emerge from this struggle.

Spaces, places and sites of waste in the city

Waste has always been directly linked to human development and to human settlements. Settlement implies accumulation, in numbers of people, their possessions and also their waste (Kennedy, 2007). Accordingly the governance of waste has always been attached to cities. The way in which waste has been managed and governed, as well as the infrastructures created to collect and transform waste have, however, changed. Municipal landfills on the edges or outskirts of urban settlements have typically been sites where waste has been disposed, dumped or buried for thousands of years, although, as Hall notes in

Chapter Two, the understanding of the value of such wastelands has changed over time to, in the present day, even being potentially valued for their ecological role. In addition, Hall also discusses the significance of the biblical traditions of wasteland and wilderness. Similarly, the religious role of wasteland is seen in Gehenna, the Jewish destination of the wicked, or hades, which was the waste yard that still exists outside Jerusalem. Gehenna was a place of constant fire caused by the burning of the corpses of animals and people, as well as waste and rubbish. In King James Bible interpretations it is translated as hell, while the term was also the basis for the name given to hell in Islam (Taylor, 2000). Simultaneous to the existence of these landfills, reusing and reducing waste have been historically ordinary practices in households (Strasser, 1999). Similarly, people have been able to discover, transform and extract the value left in waste (O'Brien, 1999, 2008). It is in the second half of the 20th century, as a result of the related processes of industrialisation, urbanisation and consumption, when households in modern societies started discarding more and more. Increasing amounts of paper, plastics or construction debris were disposed of in landfill sites.

Today a declining fraction of the waste produced in many European countries is disposed of in landfill sites where landfilling biodegradable waste has been reduced and has even disappeared in countries such as Sweden as a result of a European Union (EU) landfill directive introduced in 1999. New waste infrastructures, such as recycling stations, compost production or waste to energy incinerators, and the development of a new industrial ecology of waste marked by cradle-to-cradle thinking, coexist with traditional landfills in European countries. However, the geographies of waste infrastructures, as disclosed in this book, vary considerably within European countries where European directives are fulfilled in different ways (see, for example, Nicolli et al, 2012). Countries such as Ireland have ended up in 'waste crisis', unable to achieve the diversion policies to end biological landfilling (see, for example, Honor Fagan, 2003). This can be compared with the 'unmanagement' of waste in slums where one billion people lack sewer systems, sanitary landfills and organised formal waste collection services (UN-Habitat, 2003; Scheinberg et al, 2010).

In one way or another, with more or less frequency, with modern or traditional technology, the waste produced in cities is finally being removed. The production, collection, disposal and treatment of waste all constitute part of the essence of the cities' everyday disorganising and organising processes. The infrastructures, technologies, organisational structures, services, policies, laws and narratives created to deal with our waste have become critical to the urban condition. As unfolded in some of the chapters in this book, the utopia of the well-functioning city is only possible due to the critical urban infrastructures and services behind it (Kaika and Swyngedouw, 2000; Kaika, 2005). Simply, waste urban infrastructures (Chapter Three), waste management companies (Chapter Eight; see also Corvellec et al, 2012), householders through their recycling practices (Chapter Eleven), and even informal waste collectors (Fahmi, 2005; Fahmi and Sutton, 2006, 2010) and their 'Garbage City' make possible a functional urban life.

Interestingly, despite the criticality of waste urban infrastructures and services, these have often been taken for granted (Star, 1999). With this book we aim at gaining further understanding of these urban landscapes, infrastructures and services, 'especially when the study of urban infrastructure has been so neglected and so dominated by technical, technocratic or historical perspectives' (Graham and Marvin, 2001: 9). The study of the governance of these critical urban infrastructures has been relegated, as Graham and Marvin (2001) put it, to be the 'Cinderella' of urban studies. This has occurred for several reasons. In part it is because it has been disregarded by the social sciences, being understood as a complex and technical issue, thereby ignoring the power struggles and the questions of social and environmental justice behind them. However, also of significance is the invisibility of these infrastructures that disappear, buried in the modern city, and because of the complexity, the immensity and the boundlessness of these large technical systems with their global flows of materials and energy. All together, the result is that the study of the governance of waste has been taken for granted (Coutard et al, 2005; Guy et al, 2011).

Global waste discourses and narratives shaping local practices

Waste is a global product, produced locally, mostly in cities, and transported somewhere else, often to other locations in the same country or perhaps to developing countries where regulation is less strict with respect to how it is managed and disposed of (Honor Fagan, 2003). From this approach waste is one of the glocal metaproblems for sustainable development; it is glocal in the sense that it is a hybrid of global and local processes (Latour, 2004). Waste is, consequently, an issue of both global and local governance. This double condition implies the urgency to look at how global discourses and narratives of waste are shaping local practices, and vice versa.

Waste governance does not occur in a vacuum. Instead, it is deeply embedded in the global discourses and narratives of a sustainable development and competitiveness, material scarcity, resource use, global environmental responsibility and discourses of ecological modernisation (Davies, 2009; Davies and Mullin, 2011; see also Chapters Four and Ten). As Davies unfolds in her chapter, global narratives do not travel without incitation. Meta-organisations, such as the EU or the Organisation for Economic Co-operation and Development (OECD), drive the introduction of supranational or global narratives such as the EU Waste Hierarchy Model (European Commission, 2008) or the Integrated Solid Waste Management (ISWM), which are translated into national, regional and municipal environmental laws and policies (Davoudi, 2000, 2009). Indeed, a number of mediators are always present in all the chapters of this volume. As Latour (2005: 39) notes, mediators are understood as those who 'transform, translate, distort, and modify the meaning of the elements they are supposed to carry'. These mediators bring global narratives to local contexts, and vice versa. Consultants giving advice for the formulation of regional waste plans in Ireland, international experts supporting the local environmental movements opposed to the construction of waste incinerators in Ireland, non-governmental organisations (NGOs) promoting the exchange of experiences between informal waste collectors in the Philippines and Cairo, or even texts such as UN-Habitat's collection of best practice for waste management (UN-Habitat, 2010) are all mediators. All are more than mere intermediaries or transmitters; they make interpretations and change meanings of the models, concepts and ideas that they bring to the local practice. The final translation of global narratives varies, however. Translation of global ideas seldom implies unmediated pure diffusion (Czarniawska and Sevón, 2005). Instead, as disclosed in this book, the pre-existence of local narratives and the interpretations made by mediators and local actors shape local translations and discourses of waste and environmental governance.

Waste governance and management practices

In common with governance in other areas of sustainable development, and in particular in the context of 'sustainable cities' (Adger and Jordan, 2009), the institutional rules of the waste management sector have rapidly evolved in recent years (Davoudi and Evans, 2005). In Europe, recent changes in waste regulation, as a result of EU directives, have resulted in the commodification of waste, its transformation into a potential resource and in the creation of a market for waste (Bulkeley et al, 2007). The liberalisation of European markets for waste services to end public monopolies has not only resulted in the stimulation of a more competitive business environment, but also in the proliferation of multinational waste companies such as REMONDIS, Suez Environnement, Veolia and Waste Management Inc (as reported in various chapters in this book; see Chapters Six, Seven and Nine). In this context waste management private sector associations are lobbying to even further deregulate markets for waste services and to assume responsibility for household waste under the argument of fair competition (see Chapter Seven; see also Corvellec et al, 2012).

However, at the same time as the private sector is pushing for further deregulation of the waste services market, there are increasing political demands for environmental efficacy, particularly as a result of concerns over climate change and sustainable consumption. In Europe the adoption of the European Framework Directive on waste has resulted in new national environmental laws and waste plans which translate to national legislative and regulatory frameworks, such as the European Waste Hierarchy, to govern waste, whereby waste reduction shall have priority over recycling of materials or energy (for example, through waste incineration or waste food biogas production) (Davoudi, 2009). How this new narrative of 'wasting less' is being adopted, or in other words, how this global narrative is translated into local waste governance practices, is a question that is explored in this book (see Chapter Eight).

The influence of new public management (Hood, 1991), the privatisation of waste public companies and services, the outsourcing of public services towards public–private partnerships (PPPs) and the development of hybrid organisations (Karré, 2011; see also Chapter Seven) and other quasi-private organisations, have all favoured the hybridisation of waste management and the emergence of new actors such as waste incineration companies or citizens' recycling cooperatives (see Chapter Ten) to collect and handle household solid waste. The nature of these public–private hybrid waste management companies and their consequences for citizens, private waste operators, its political governance and internal staff also unfolds in this book. The contradictions faced in governing these hybrid organisations, such as balancing profitability with environmental protection, or the difficulties in politically governing a critical highly technological infrastructure (Davoudi, 2006; Thomasson, 2009), are discussed in Chapter Seven.

Furthermore, in Europe the EU 'has been able to exert strong environmental control since the late 1980s' (Davoudi, 2009: 138). Since the 1990s the majority of environmental regulatory measures introduced in European countries have originated in EU initiatives, including waste. The EU Waste Framework Directive (1999/31/

EC; see Council of the European Communities, 1999) and more recent legislation has been very influential in terms of its impact on emerging national, regional and local policies, discourses and narratives of waste. As a result, waste governance is no longer an exclusive responsibility of the city authorities. Rather, it takes place in the framework of the network society (Castells, 1996) through multilevel network governance (Bache and Flinders, 2004). The responsibility for waste is, in most countries today, shared among many parties. For example, a producer responsibility system has been set up since the mid-1990s in European countries such as Sweden or Denmark, for packaging, tyres, newsprint, end-of-life vehicles and waste electrical and electronic equipment. The management of industrial waste has been handed over to the market in most European countries, and so has the management of dangerous waste. However, many municipalities still retain responsibility for household waste (and industrial waste of a similar kind) within the limit of their jurisdiction, which at times may put them into commercial and regulatory conflict with transnational waste corporations, a number of which, perhaps ironically, had their origins in municipal waste bodies.

In this volume Minervini (Chapter Six) describes the multilevel governance of waste when he narrates the journey of his bottle of wine from his bin, to the glass recycling container and finally into the hands of a multinational corporation thousands of kilometres away from the place where its content was consumed. A myriad of institutions and organisations populate the complex organising of waste in and out of our cities, replacing 'predictable and monolithic monopolies with highly fragmented and differentiated styles of service provision with highly complex, and often hidden, geometries and geographies' (Graham and Marvin, 2001: 14). The multilevel governance of waste reveals interesting aspects such as the geographies of waste governance (Davies, 2008), whereby flows of goods and waste are constantly on the move, crossing national boundaries driven by market rules. Italian waste is incinerated in the Netherlands; European fragments of electronic waste are transported overseas to African and Chinese landfill sites; and recyclable materials recovered in Nicaragua by scavengers are exported to Central America, China and even Europe via Spain (Zapata Campos and Zapata, 2012).

Waste and environmental, economic and social justice

Multilevel governance links 'the policy-making processes of supranational, national and sub-national public agencies and, to a lesser degree, non-public organizations' (Bovaird, 2005: 219). Since governance refers to the interactions between civil society and governments, it is crucial to explore how communities are not only the mere object of waste policies and global discourses, but civil society also has the capacity to contest and influence waste public policies, and with a degree of success. As some of the contributions to this book prove, the lack of citizen participation, or the incapability of states and local governments to understand the local needs, interests and narratives of society and nature, can turn into potential grievances in the waste policies formulation and implementation stages (see, for example, Chapter Ten, this volume). Local protests against the allocation of landfill sites or waste incinerators have turned into environmental campaigns whereby links are made between local waste crisis and global environmental concerns and movements (see Chapter Ten; see also Honor Fagan, 2003). Similarly, communities of informal waste collectors around the world have enacted episodes of community mobilisation and struggle against state waste privatisation policies (such as those presented in Chapter Nine). Because waste is an accessible asset for poor communities, the commoditisation and privatisation of former municipal waste collection services has turned out to be a threat for the livelihood of microentrepreneurs and their families.

The design of waste policies and plans and the enactment of 'sustainable' waste governance is not an easy task. As Bell and Sweeting emphasise in Chapter Eleven, waste policies have often failed to understand the heterogeneity of cities and their dwellers, resulting in issues of environmental injustice (Bulkeley and Gregson, 2009). New waste governance and practices imply the transformation of citizens into active participants in the waste management system (Bulkeley et al, 2007). Recycling systems at source are based on the active role of householders to classify and separate waste into different categories. The production of household waste is the result of social lifestyles, income, education and other cultural and environmental values. In many cases the consumer is being encouraged to actively be involved in assisting the development of the waste market under the guise of helping the environment. Waste urban infrastructures perform as a mirror of society (Chapter Three), meaning that waste flows and its composition and volume vary according to sociotechnical changes. While in Managua

70 per cent of its waste was organic due to lower levels of consumption and industrialisation, in Gothenburg the consumption of electronic products and the subsequent disposal of electronic waste is increasing dramatically, year on year.

In Chapter Eleven Bell and Sweeting call our attention to how there may be more need for waste collection in deprived areas because often more people live in each household, there is a greater use of cheaper and more heavily packaged food, household items may be of inferior quality and, therefore, not last as long, and because poorer people are less likely to have a car with which to dispose of items themselves (Hastings, 2007). In other words, waste services have to be appropriate to the local context. Otherwise, new regimes, that is, new modes of waste governance such as 'landfilling less' (Chapter Eight) and the promotion of recycling, can 'come at a cost to some of the households least able to bear it' in the global North (see Chapter Eleven). National and municipal waste policies have typically failed to contemplate issues of environmental injustice when designing these policies, as demonstrated in the case of the less well-off areas of Bristol. Instead, pressure on households, rather than business, is a result of a policy framework that favours recycling rather than the reduction of waste (see Chapter Eleven). As Bell and Sweeting point out, EU legislation introduced at the end of the 1990s (The Packaging Waste Directive 94/62/EC; see Council of the European Communities, 1994) requires packaging to be minimised and to be designed for recovery and reuse. However, in most European countries waste directives and practice have focused on recovery, rather than reduction. In Sweden the National Federation of Waste Packaging has long been criticised by municipalities for not meeting their goals to reduce waste (Swedish Waste Management, 2011). It is estimated that one quarter to one third of domestic waste in the UK is made up of packaging (The Open University, 2008), and householders are carrying the burden of disposing of packaging that is produced to increase business sales. As Bell and Sweeting (Chapter Eleven) report, 'this is clear injustice, with commercial interests benefiting at the cost of householders.' In other words, although waste prevention is in the discourse of national waste policies, in practice waste packaging increases, as a business, and at the costs of citizens, and especially of citizens in less well-off areas.

Indeed, a major theme in several chapters in this book is that waste policies designed to reduce environmental degradation can be paradoxically counter-productive when they ignore the complexity and heterogeneity of cities. In some income-deprived areas in Bristol, or in the informal settlements in Managua, residents lit fires in order to dispose of waste and to avoid paying for it. In the informal settlements, both in Managua and Cairo, modern waste trucks could not get into the narrow streets of the informal city, leaving an important part of the city out of the formal waste management system, resulting in illegal dumping. The governance of urban informality (Roy and Alsayyad, 2004) therefore becomes critical for the governance of socioenvironmental issues such as waste.

Structure of the book

Part I introduces the study of waste infrastructures and places in the city. In Chapter Two, Michael Hall explores the significance of 'drosscapes' (Berger, 2006), and the different understandings of city and suburban wastelands. He highlights how such wastelands may, in fact, be ecologically rich and important for the conservation of biodiversity and even endangered species. He also draws parallels between contemporary urban understandings of wasteland to historical notions of wasteland and its importance for conservation. In Chapter Three, María José Zapata Campos uses the notion of heterotopia (Foucault, 1986) to rethink the functions and meanings of waste urban infrastructures, based on narratives of waste from the cities of Managua in Nicaragua and Gothenburg in Sweden. Based on her ethnographic research, she explores how, by isolating and hiding waste, waste infrastructures make possible the utopia of a well-functioning city. She also discusses how efficient waste infrastructures can contribute to hide the consequences of the consumption and discard society by obscuring the link between consumption and the increasing overflow of waste.

Part II provides rich illustrations of how global narratives are locally translated into practice, covering global waste narratives such as ISWH or Zero Waste. In Chapter Four, Anna Davies adopts a comparative governance framework to explore evolving narratives of municipal solid waste policy in Ireland and New Zealand through an examination of policy interventions, stakeholder interactions and outcomes. She undertakes a detailed analysis of global waste governance narratives and their influence over national and regional waste policies, policy mechanisms such as targets, levies and charges, and waste management outcomes. In Chapter Five, Patrik Zapata explores the translation of global narratives of waste management formulated by UN-Habitat into local waste practices in Managua, Nicaragua. Excerpts of two documents produced by UN-Habitat related to sustainable waste management are analysed. Inspired by deconstruction methods (Martin, 1990), Zapata traces how, why and by whom these narratives have been translated, and which ones have been stabilised as the predominant narratives in the discourse of a sustainable waste management.

Part III outlines the practices of governing waste in contemporary cities. The three chapters in this section tackle issues of multilevel environmental governance, the regionalisation of waste management, privatisation and the marketisation of formerly municipally owned waste management companies into hybrid municipal solid waste management companies. Waste governance and management practices are also related to the introduction of ambitious narratives of 'wasting less'. Using actor-network theory (ANT) (Callon, 1986; Latour, 1987; Law and Hassard, 1998), in Chapter Six Dario Minervini describes how waste governance and policies are translated into sociotechnical practices. Based on ethnographic research, Minervini shadows his own wine bottle and narrates its journey from the container collected by the regional waste management company in Molfetta, southern Italy, until it becomes part of the glass purchased by a multinational corporation. In Chapter Seven, Philip Karré examines how, as a result of processes of privatisation, deregulation and marketisation, public services such as waste management have been outsourced to public waste management organisations. As a result, municipal waste services have evolved either to behave like companies through hybrid public waste companies, or to be sold off to the private sector, often to multinational corporations. By taking the Dutch waste management sector as an example, Karré addresses what hybridity in waste management means, how it manifests and what opportunities and dilemmas it raises. In Chapter Eight, Hervé Corvellec and Johan Hultman demonstrate, based on the case of a Swedish municipal waste management company, that waste management companies participate in a decisive manner to the design of the sociomateriality of waste, and that this participation gives them a particularly important role for urban development. They describe three successive waste governance regimes – a landfilling regime, a less landfilling regime and a wasting less regime – based on the Swedish waste management case, and explain how each entails a specific sociomateriality of waste.

Part IV deals with the role of civil society in the governance of waste. The chapters in this section shift the focus to look at citizens as something other than the mere objects of policies and narratives of waste. City dwellers become informal waste collectors, members of environmental movements or active householders exhorted to classify the increasing amount of waste packaging. In Chapter Nine, Wael Fahmi and Keith Sutton focus on the impacts of waste privatisation policies of solid waste management on local informal waste collectors in Cairo and the 'garbage city', by employing narratives of waste collectors. They deal with narratives of community mobilisation and the struggle against state waste governance policies. They describe how a potential local–global partnership between local Zabaleens and the international waste corporations contracted by the city did not prove fruitful because of power asymmetries. Despite the loss of waste assets on behalf of local waste collectors, the authors place the Zabaleens' narrative as a not-ended story, and frame it in a context of radical policy action and major political events that might change the techno-institutional order in Egypt in which waste governance is embedded. In Chapter Ten, Liam Leonard examines the tensions between the policy discourse of ecological modernisation, through the Irish state's regional waste plans, the potential construction of waste incineration facilities, and the local narratives surrounding the mobilisation processes of community movements. He describes how community mobilisation and environmental movements have successfully introduced recycling practices and challenged concepts of industrial growth and ecological modernisation. Chapter Eleven is based on narratives of waste collected from neighbours in a community in Bristol; it provides evidence of unequal and unjust burdens faced by deprived communities in relation to waste collection services. The chapter makes a particular contribution to the literature on waste from the discipline of social policy, a field of study that has lagged behind the environmental debate despite the obvious links between the environment and poverty.

In the concluding chapter there is a summary of the key themes and findings emerging from the book, with a focus on how global narratives are translated into local waste practices and the consequences of this for the organising of waste in cities. The transition towards 'wasting less' narratives and governance is discussed. From this, implications of power, environmental justice and an urban sustainable development are drawn for future waste policy governance.

As noted at the start of this chapter, this volume offers a contemporary critical social sciences perspective on the issue of organising waste in cities that has often been positioned in economic-technical discourses. It emphasises the way in which the notion of waste and the narratives and discourses associated with it are socially constructed. Such an observation has profound implications for the governance of waste and the local waste handling practices, and therefore the 'traditional' engineering and economic discourses of urban waste management. However, as illustrated throughout the book, waste policies, although well meaning, that do not understand and engage with the social context within which they are or will become embedded may be doomed to failure, or partial success at best. Given the environmental necessity of improving urban waste management's contribution to lessening the impact of cities on climate change, it therefore becomes imperative that disciplinary boundaries and silos with respect to waste management be bridged. We hope that this book will make a contribution to this task.

References

Adger, N. and Jordan, A. (2009) *Governing sustainability*, Cambridge: Cambridge University Press.

Bache, I. and Flinders, M. (2004) *Multi-level governance*, Oxford: Oxford University Press.

Barton, J.B., Dalley, D. and Patel, V.S. (1996) 'Life cycle assessment for waste management', *Waste Management*, vol 16, nos 1-3, pp 35-50.

Berger, A. (2006) *Drosscape: Wasting land in urban America*, New York: Princeton Architectural Press.

Bovaird, T. (2005) 'Public governance: balancing stakeholder power in a network society', *International Review of Administrative Sciences*, vol 71, pp 217-28.

Bulkeley, H. and Gregson, N. (2009) 'Crossing the threshold: municipal waste policy and household waste generation', *Environment and Planning A*, vol 41, 929-45.

Bulkeley, H. and Watson, M. (2007) 'Modes of governing municipal waste', *Environment and Planning A*, vol 39, pp 2733-53.

Callon, M. (1986) 'Some elements of a sociology of translation: Domestication of the scallops and the fishermen of St Brieuc Bay', in J. Law (ed) *Power, action and belief*, London: Routledge & Kegan Paul, pp 196-223.

Castells, M. (1996) *The rise of the network society*, Malden, MA: Blackwell.

Cooper, T. (2009) 'War on waste? The politics of waste and recycling in post-war Britain, 1950-1975', *Capitalism Nature Socialism*, vol 20, no 4, pp 53-72.

Council of the European Communities (1994) *European Parliament and Council Directive 94/62/EC of 20 December 1994 on packaging and packaging waste*, Brussels: Council of the European Communities.

Council of the European Communities (1999) *Council Directive 1999/31/EC of 26 April 1999 on the landfill of waste*, Brussels: Council of the European Communities.

Corvellec, H. and Hultman, J. (2012) 'From "less landfilling" to "wasting less". Societal narratives, socio-materiality, and organizations', *Journal of Organizational Change Management*, vol 25, no 2, pp 297-314.

Corvellec, H., Bramryd, T. and Hultman, J. (2012) 'The business model of solid waste management in Sweden – a case study of two municipally-owned companies', *Waste Management and Research*, vol 30, no 5, pp 512-18.

Coutard, O., Hanley, R.E. and Zimmermann, R. (2005) *Sustaining urban networks: The social diffusion of large technical systems*, Abingdon: Routledge.

Czarniawska, B. (2004) *Narratives in social science research*, London: Sage Publications.

Czarniawska, B. and Sevón, G. (2005) *Global ideas: How ideas, objects and practices travel in the global economy*, Malmö: Liber & Copenhagen Business School Press.

Davies, A. (2008) *Geographies of garbage governance: Interventions, interactions and outcomes*, Aldershot: Ashgate.

Davies, A. (2009) 'Clean and green? A governance analysis of waste management in New Zealand', *Journal of Environmental Planning and Management*, vol 52, no 2, pp 157-77.

Davies, A. and Mullin, S. (2011) 'Greening the economy: interrogating sustainability innovations beyond the mainstream', *Journal of Economic Geography*, vol 11, no 5, pp 793-816.

Davoudi, S. (2000) 'Planning for waste management: changing discourses and institutional relationships', *Progress in Planning*, vol 53, pp 165-216.

Davoudi, S. (2006) 'Evidence-policy interface in strategic waste planning in urban environment: the "technical" and the "social"', *Environment and Planning C: Government and Policy*, vol 24, no 5, pp 681-700.

Davoudi, S. (2009) 'Governing waste: introduction to this special issue', *Journal of Environmental Planning and Management*, vol 52, no 2, pp 131-6.

Davoudi, S. and Evans, N. (2005) 'The challenge of governance in regional waste planning', *Environment and Planning C: Government and Policy*, vol 23, no 4, pp 493-519.

Douglas, M. (1966) *Purity and danger: An analysis of the concepts of pollution and taboo*, London: Routledge.

European Commission (2008) 'Directive 2008/98/EC of the European Parliament and the Council on waste and repealing', *Official Journal of the European Union L 312/3*, Brussels: European Commission.

Fahmi, W. (2005) 'The impact of privatization of solid waste management on the Zabaleen garbage collectors of Cairo', *Environment and Urbanization*, vol 17, no 2, pp 155-70.

Fahmi, W. and Sutton, K. (2006) 'Cairo's Zabaleen garbage recyclers: Multi-nationals' takeover and state relocation plans', *Habitat International,* vol 30, no 4, pp 809-37.

Fahmi, W. and Sutton, K. (2010) 'Cairo's contested garbage: Sustainable solid waste management and the Zabaleen's right to the city', *Sustainability*, vol 2, pp 1765-83.

Foote, S. and Mazzolini, E. (eds) (2012) *Histories of the dustheap: Waste, material cultures, social justice*, Cambridge, MA: The MIT Press.

Foucault, M. (1986) 'Of other spaces', *Diacritics*, vol 16, pp 22-7.

Fried, J. and Eyles, J. (2011) 'Welcome waste – interpreting narratives of radioactive waste disposal in two small towns in Ontario, Canada', *Journal of Risk Research*, vol 14, no 9, pp 1017-37.

Graham, S. and Marvin, S. (2001) *Splintering urbanism: Networked infrastructures, technological mobilities and the urban condition*, London: Routledge.

Gregson, N. (2009) 'Recycling as policy and assemblage', *Geography*, vol 94, no 1, pp 61-5.

Gregson, N. and Crang, M. (2010) 'Materiality and waste: Inorganic vitality in a networked world', *Environment and Planning A*, vol 42, pp 1026-32.

Guy, S., Marvin, S., Medd, W. and Moss, T. (2011) *Shaping urban infrastructures: Intermediaries and the governance of socio-technical networks*, London: Earthscan.

Hastings, A. (2007) 'Territorial justice and neighbourhood environmental services: a comparison of provision to deprived and better off neighbourhoods in the UK', *Environment and Planning C: Government and Policy*, vol 25, no 6, pp 896-917.

Hawkins, G. (2006) *The ethics of waste: How we relate to rubbish*, Lanham, MD: Rowman & Littlefield.

Hawkins, G. (2009) 'The politics of bottled water: Assembling bottled water as brand, waste and oil', *Journal of Cultural Economy*, vol 2, nos 1-2, pp 183-95.

Hawkins, G. (2010) 'Plastic materialities', in B. Braun and S.J. Whatmore (eds) *Political matter: Technoscience, democracy, and public life*, Minneapolis, MN: University of Minnesota Press, pp 119-38.

Honor Fagan, G. (2003) 'Sociological reflections on governing waste', *Irish Journal of Sociology*, vol 12, no 1, pp 67-84.

Hood, C. (1991) 'A public management for all seasons?', *Public Administration*, vol 69, no 1, pp 3-19.

Hultman, J. and Corvellec, H. (2012) 'The waste hierarchy model: from the socio-materiality of waste to a politics of consumption', *Environment and Planning A*, vol 44, no 10, pp 2413- 27.

Hung, M.-L., Ma, H. and Yang, W.-F. (2007) 'A novel sustainable decision making model for municipal solid waste management', *Waste Management*, vol 27, no 2, pp 209-19.

Kaika, M. (2005) *City of flows: Modernity, nature, and the city*, New York: Routledge.

Kaika, M. and Swyngedouw, E. (2000) 'Fetishizing the modern city: The phantasmagoria of urban technological networks', *International Journal of Urban and Regional Research*, vol 24, no 1, 120-38.

Karré, P.M. (2011) *Heads and tails: Both sides of the coin. An analysis of hybrid organizations in the Dutch waste management sector*, The Hague: Eleven International Publishing.

Kennedy, G. (2007) *An ontology of trash*, New York: State University of New York.

Lane, R. and Gorman-Murray, A. (eds) (2011) *Material geographies of the household*, Aldershot: Ashgate.

Latour, B. (1987) *Science in action: How to follow scientists and engineers through society*, Milton Keynes: Open University Press.

Latour, B. (2004) 'On the difficulty of being glocal', *Domus*, no 2, March.

Latour, B. (2005) *Reassembling the social: An introduction to actor-network-theory*, Oxford: Oxford University Press.

Law, J. and Hassard, J. (1999) *Actor-network theory and after*, Oxford: Blackwell.

MacIntyre, A. (1981) *After virtue*, London: Duckworth.

MacKillop, F. (2009) 'The construction of "waste" in the UK steel industry', *Journal of Environmental Planning and Management*, vol 52, no 2, pp 177-94.

Martin, J. (1990) 'Deconstructing organizational taboos: the suppression of gender conflict in organizations', *Organization Science*, vol 1, no 4, pp 339-59.

Morrissey, A.J. and Browne, J. (2004) 'Waste management models and their application to sustainable waste management', *Waste Management*, vol 24, no 3, pp 297-308.

Nicolli, F., Mazzanti, M. and Iafolla, V. (2012) 'Waste dynamics, country heterogeneity and European environmental policy effectiveness', *Journal of Environmental Policy & Planning*, vol 14, no 4, 371-93.

O'Brien, M. (1999) 'Rubbish-power: towards a sociology of the rubbish society', in J. Hearn and S. Roseneil (eds) *Consuming cultures: Power and resistance*, Explorations in Sociology, vol 55, London: Macmillan, pp 262-77.

O'Brien, M. (2008) *A crisis of waste? Understanding the rubbish society*, New York: Routledge.

Open University, The (2008) *The Open University household waste study: Key findings for 2007*, London: Department for Environment, Food and Rural Affairs.

Robinson, J. (2006) *Ordinary cities: Between modernity and development*, London: Routledge.

Roy, A. and Alsayyad, N. (2004) *Urban informality*, Oxford: Lexington.

Scheinberg, A., Wilson, D.C. and Rodic-Wiersma, L. (2010) *Solid waste management in the world's cities: Water and sanitation in the world's cities 2010*, London: UN-Habitat/Earthscan.

Skordilis, A. (2004) 'Modelling of integrated solid waste management systems in an island', *Resources, Conservation and Recycling*, vol 41, no 3, pp 243-54.

Star, S. (1999) 'The ethnography of infrastructure', *American Behavioral Scientist*, vol 43, pp 377-91.

Strasser, S. (1999) *Waste and want: A social history of trash*, New York: Metropolitan Books.

Swedish Waste Management (2011) 'Waste Sweden' (www.avfallsverige.se).

Taylor, R.P. (2000) *Death and the afterlife: A cultural encyclopedia*, Santa Barbara, CA: ABC-CLIO.

Thomasson, A. (2009) *Navigating the landscape of ambiguity: A stakeholder approach to the governance and management of hybrid organisations*, Lund: Lund Business Press.

Tuler, S. and Webler, T. (2010) 'How preferences for public participation are linked to perceptions of the context, preferences for outcomes, and individual characteristics', *Environmental Management*, vol 46, no 2, 254-67.

UN-Habitat (2003) *The challenge of slums: Global reports on human settlements 2003*, London: Earthscan and UN-Habitat Settlements Programme.

UN-Habitat (2010) *Solid waste management in the world's cities*, London: Earthscan.

Zapata Campos, M.J. and Zapata, P. (2012) 'Changing La Chureca. Organising city resilience through action nets', *Journal of Change Management*, vol 12, no 3, pp 323-37.

Part I

Spaces, places and sites of waste in the city

TWO

The ecological and environmental significance of urban wastelands and drosscapes

C. Michael Hall

Introduction

Waste is a major theme in urban planning and landscape design. However, while the majority of chapters in this book focus on urban waste in the form of household and industrial waste, this chapter examines waste and more particularly wastelands in the urban spatial context. Waste is a difficult concept to define yet, as Blaustein (2011: 5) observes, 'our cultural definitions and regulations of waste are central to the ordering of our environments and ourselves' (see also Kennedy, 2007). Blaustein (2011: 5) argues that ideas of waste are 'registered in terms of space (blight, sprawl, vacancy), time (waiting, boredom, drudgery), resources (refuse, trash), and increasingly in terms of digital information technologies (e-waste, obsolescence, "delete"), waste marks the residue, the left-over, the cast-off, the remainder, the damaged, the unclassifiable, the useless'. According to Lynch (1990a: 146), waste 'is worthless or unused for human purpose. It is a lessening of something without useful result; it is loss and abandonment, decline, separation and death. It is the spent and valueless material left after some act of production or consumption, but can also refer to any used thing: garbage, trash, litter, junk, impurity and dirt. There are waste things, waste lands, waste time and wasted lives.' Similarly, Berger (2006a: 203) argues that:

> contemporary modes of industrial production driven by economical and consumerist influences contribute to urbanization and the formation of waste landscapes – meaning actual *waste* (such as municipal solid waste, sewage, scrap metal, and so on), *wasted* places (such as abandoned and/or contaminated sites) or *wasteful* places (such as

> oversized parking lots or duplicate big-box retail venues). (emphasis in original)

The description of parts of the city as wasteland is often seen in terms of the social construction of the urban environment (Hough, 2004). While such a perspective is important for understanding how landscapes are perceived, it may tell us little about the urban ecological significance of such locations. This chapter provides an ecological perspective on supposed urban wastelands by identifying their environmental functions. It first examines the way in which wasteland has come to be regarded as urban wilderness, before looking at issues of urban biodiversity. It then discusses the ecological value of wastelands that are some of the most species-rich environments in many cities. However, although ecologically significant, wasteland is not necessarily socially valued. The chapter concludes by noting the importance of linking the ways in which our understanding of what constitutes urban wasteland are socially and environmentally constructed, and its significance for urban ecology.

Wasteland as urban wilderness

Berger (2006a), like other commentators (see, for example, Lynch, 1972, 1990a, 1990b; Jakle and Wilson, 1992; Southworth, 2001), regards wasteland as intrinsic to urban development, particularly in the US. 'The processes of urban wasting operate throughout the metropolis, from center to edge, and at multiple scales' (Southworth, 2001: 5). This is partly the result of the dynamics of urban growth, with urban cores and inner cities declining in value as the growth edge of the city advances in rapid horizontal urbanisation ('urban sprawl'), and after economic and production regimes have ended, and as a result of mobility and relatively low transportation costs (Berger, 2006a, 2006b). However, according to Berger (2006a), the creation of wasteland as a result of such processes should not be seen as a negative, as 'from its deindustrializing inner core to its sprawling periphery to the transitional landscapes in between, the city is a manifestation of industrial processes that naturally produce waste' (2006a: 1999). Instead, waste landscapes are often 'an indicator of healthy urban growth' (Berger, 2006a: 203). However, Berger acknowledges that such understandings are not shared by many urban dwellers.

Similarly, the ambivalence towards wasteland, as towards wilderness (Hall and Frost, 2009), is to be found in non-Anglo-American landscape traditions. Erz (1992: 3) noted that there has always existed a dualism about having any kind of wasteland in German environmental thought: 'On the one hand, its appearance is considered non-acceptable by some

– a sentiment based, in my opinion, on the typical German attitudes of orderliness, cleanliness, and ... "civic beauty". On the other hand, wasteland has provoked an appreciation of romantic beauty and a fanciful enthusiasm for wilderness.'

Berger (2006s, 2006b) developed a new term, 'drosscape', to describe the in-between nature of waste landscapes. The term implies 'that dross, or waste, is scaped, or resurfaced/reinscribed, by new human intentions ... shared origins with the words *waste* and *vast*, two terms frequently used to describe the contemporary nature of horizontal urbanization, as well as connections to the words *vanity*, *vain*, and *vacant*, all of which relate to waste through the form of empty gestures' (Berger, 2006a: 210, emphasis in original). In order to survive, drosscapes are regarded as dependent on the production of waste landscapes from other types of urban development. 'In this rubric one may describe drosscaping as a sort of scavenging of the city surface for interstitial landscape remains' (Berger, 2006a: 210). Nevertheless, as degraded and interstitial entities, 'drosscapes have few caretakers, guardians, or spokespersons. The importance of a drosscape is only appreciated through a bottom-up advocacy process' (Berger, 2006a: 213).

The concept of wasteland is one that resonates strongly in contemporary urban studies. Wasteland has been seen as an example of Foucault's (1998) notion of heterotopia, a range of 'different spaces' and 'other spaces' that somehow challenge or contest the space we live in (see Johnson, 2006; Dehaene and de Cauter, 2008). Terms that surround the concept of wasteland include 'dead zones' (Doron, 2000, 2008), 'free space' (Boffet and Rocca Serra, 2001), 'nameless space' (Boeri, 1993; Eshel, 2003), 'blank space' (Jackson, 1997), 'brown fields' (Bowman and Pagano, 2000; Haase, 2008), 'liminal space' (Endsjø, 2000), 'no man's land' (Woods, 2000), 'derelict land' (Oxenham, 1966), 'urban void' (Cheung, 2000; Clapp, 2005), 'terrain vague' (de Sola-Morales, 1995), 'untended landscapes' (Lynch, 1990a), 'blight' (Greenberg and Schneider, 1996), 'industrial ruins' (Edensor, 2005), 'urban desert' (Guttenberg, 1978), 'backsides' (Lynch, 1990a, 1990b), 'brownscape' (Berger, 2008; Grimm and Dosch, 2010), 'gapscape' (Hormigo and Morita, 2004), 'drosscape' (Berger 2006a) and 'edgeland' (Farley and Roberts, 2011). As Doron (2008: 203) points out, 'The multiplicity of names and some of their meanings, show the difficulty in defining those spaces.'

Haid (2011), for example, understood urban wasteland as a form of interstitial wilderness with its spontaneous growth of vegetation. Neither cultivated nor wild, Haid regarded these areas as hybridised heterotopias where the heterotopic qualities of these landscapes counterpoint a commodified abstract public space and strengthen a more desirable differential space where hybridity and amalgamations are dominating and appreciated. Although not adopting Haid's theoretical stance, Farley and Roberts (2011: 26) regard 'edgelands' as England's true wilderness: 'We know that an unseen, untouched English landscape is a myth. We know that a long and complex interaction between constant natural processes and more recent human activity has largely formed all the landscapes we can see today, and that landscape is indivisible from the human world.' In such places nature, if allowed, reoccupies the built environment. For example, in referring to Bidston Moss on the Wirral, Farley and Roberts observe:

> … a dark waste ground beneath the flyovers … it seems as if every colour and variety of polyethylene, polypropylene, polystyrene and polyvinyl has landed here … it's a huge litter trap, an open space surrounded by people passing through very quickly, an unacknowledged or quickly disregarded blindspot. Looking closer, you can see how truefoils and bindweeds have begun to grow back over some of the takeaway cartons and soft-drinks bottles. (Farley and Roberts, 2011: 35)

Indeed, wasteland as urban wilderness is a recurring theme in studies of wasteland (Lynch, 1972), and represents a fundamental change in understandings of wilderness given that historically wilderness and the city have usually been represented as opposites (Nash, 1982; Hall, 1992; Zeveloff et al, 1992; Lerup, 2006), although this spatial shift in understandings of wilderness does recall Tuan's observation on wilderness in the late 20th century that 'As a state of the mind, true wilderness exists only in the great sprawling cities' (Tuan, 1974: 112). Nevertheless, wastelands as wilderness play a major role, not only in understanding the cultural values of wasteland with respect to its otherness and even counter-institutional role, but also attitudes towards the natural environment. According to Lynch (1990a: 153):

> Wastelands are the havens of rebellious, marginal, illegal people. Swamps were the hideouts of the southern slaves and the refuge of the Cajuns. Mountains harbored the Cuban guerrillas, and the displaced intellectuals of China. The cold, wet, northern margins of European Russia were peopled by Old Believers, in flight from the Tatars and religious heresy. Wastelands are places of despair, but they also shield relicts, and the first weak forms of some new thing, a new religion,

a new politics. They are places for dreams, for antisocial acts, for exploration and growth.

To the English translators of the King James Bible, wilderness had a central position as both a descriptive and a symbolic concept. To the ancient Hebrews wilderness was an environment of evil in which the wasteland was identified with God's curse. Paradise, or Eden, was the antithesis of wilderness. There is the story of Adam and Eve's dismissal from the Garden of Eden, from a watered, lush paradise to a 'cursed' land of 'thorns and thistles' (*Genesis* 2:4). The experience of the Israelites during the Exodus added another dimension to the Judeo-Christian attitude towards wilderness. For 40 years the Jews, led by Moses, wandered in the 'howling waste of the wilderness' (*Deuteronomy* 32:10) that was the Sinai Peninsula (Funk, 1959).

The fact that land came to be seen as waste paradoxically came to play a critical role in its conservation (Hall and Frost, 2009). For example, the majority of North Americans saw the land as something to be conquered and made productive. The first reservations for the preservation of scenery tended to be established in areas that were judged to be wastelands that had no economic value in terms of agriculture, grazing, lumbering or mining (Runte, 1972; Hall, 1989). According to Runte (1973: 5):

> An abundance of public land that seemed worthless – not environmental concern or aesthetic appreciation – made possible the establishment of most national parks in the United States. Nothing else can explain how aesthetic conservationists, who in the past have represented only a small minority of Americans, were able to achieve some success in a nation dominated by a firm commitment to industrial achievement and the exploitation of resources. A surplus of marginal public land enabled the United States to "afford" aesthetic conservation; national parks protected only such areas as were considered valueless for profitable lumbering, mining, grazing, or agriculture. Indeed, throughout the history of the national parks, the concept of "useless" scenery has virtually determined which areas the nation would protect and how it would protect them.

In the Australian and New Zealand context, if land was 'unused', it was regarded as waste (Ramson, 1991; Hall, 1989, 1992). In New South Wales 'Crown leases and conditions of purchase of Crown land, required the former to ringbark or clear all standing timber. In some areas this meant destruction of valuable timber trees, in others, stimulation of soil erosion, and in all areas, tremendous losses of wildlife thus bereft of habitat and cover' (Strom, 1979: 45). Similarly to the US the perception of land as waste played a critical role in having land set aside for scenic conservation in Australia and New Zealand. For example, under the Tasmanian Waste Lands Act 1863 and the subsequent Crown Lands Act a variety of reserves were established for their scenic value (Hall, 1992).

One of the key lessons of the role of wasteland in natural area conservation is that wilderness is still seen by many people as waste or worthless land that needs to be made productive, for example, by tourism (Runte, 1973; Hall, 1989; Frost and Hall, 2009), in order to assign it a value. As Haid (2011) noted with respect to urban wastelands, these areas offer high degrees of biodiversity and are habitats for wild animals and therefore important factors in seeking to render cities more ecologically sustainable. However, wild and unmaintained nature is often considered unattractive and opposed to prevailing concepts of homogeneous spaces shaped by capitalism. This aesthetic notion is well established, for example, with respect to the notion of 'derelict' land. As Barr (1969: 14) states, 'To most of us "derelict land" means virtually any land which is ugly or unattractive in appearance.' Lynch (1990a) similarly suggested that waste can be useful, but what it is lacking is not necessarily use value, but exchange value on the capitalist market. Dereliction, Lynch points out, is always in relation to the market. 'If it pays, it isn't derelict. If it doesn't pay, due to some human devilment, and once did pay, then it is derelict' (Lynch, 1990a: 98). 'Those marvellous empty zones' of Doron (2008) are therefore not so marvellous as to be prized for their ecological values. Yet, as the next section discusses, wastelands can have substantial environmental roles and values that may serve as the basis for more sustainable cities.

Urban biodiversity

Cities are not usually thought of as important for biodiversity, although the importance of urban biodiversity conservation is increasingly recognised (Müller et al, 2010). Davies et al (2011) note that a relative lack of research on the ecosystem services that urban areas provide is a legacy of the perception that urban ecosystems have limited ecological value because they are heavily modified by humans and relatively small in size (see also Puth and Burns, 2009; Del Tredici, 2010). Yet, several authors have found that urban areas often contain more plant species than rural areas (see, for example, Walters, 1970; Pysek, 1989);

this is especially the case with respect to non-native species. A strong positive relationship has also been demonstrated between the number of vascular plant species and the population size of cities, and a weaker positive relationship with city size. In small and medium-sized towns, between 530 and 560 species of ferns and flowering plants are usually found. Between 650 and 730 species are found in cities with 100,000 to 200,000 inhabitants, 900 and 1,000 species in cities with populations ranging from 250,000 to 400,000, and in cities with more than a million inhabitants, the number of species usually exceeds 1,300 (Klotz, 1990; Pysek, 1993). There are several reasons for this:

- urban areas provide extremely heterogeneous habitats;
- urban areas are focal points for the introduction of new species as a result of trade, transport and tourism connections;
- they are locations in their own right for the evolution of new taxa as a result of isolation, hybridisation and introgression; and
- their relationship to their surrounding area may also influence the number of species in the city.

London provides a useful example of the range of habitats available in large cities. Of the Greater London area of nearly 158,000 hectares, two thirds are occupied by green open space and water, and nearly one fifth is considered valuable wildlife habitat. Nature conservation designations apply to approximately 16 per cent of this area, covering a range of habitats, many of which would be regarded as derelict land, including wetlands, urban woodland, water bodies, heathland, rail sides, urban wasteland, marshes and mudflats (Wilby and Perry, 2006). However, although London's wasteland is recognised as being ecologically significant, its status means that its overall contribution to biodiversity conservation, at least by area covered, is hard to assess. For example, in the case of London, while it is recognised that there are over 1,000 hectares of railway land, line sides and road sides alone that fulfils criteria of sites of importance for nature conservation, the area of wasteland is unknown because of definitional issues as well as redevelopment. In addition, there are 31,000 hectares of gardens, 1,300 hectares of cemeteries and churchyards, 273 hectares of marshland and 80 hectares of heathland (Wilby and Perry, 2006).

Yet cities are heterogeneous in space and time and are highly dynamic spaces. Biodiversity richness is not evenly distributed across the urban landscape. Different densities of buildings act as a major driver of plant species composition. Increased density has a strong negative influence on species richness mainly because it tends to generate higher temperatures compared to more open areas (Godefroid and Koedam, 2007).

Wasteland and urban species richness

Although mainly responsible for species richness in wasteland in cities, 'the abandoned rural landscape which consists of marginal or degraded urban land that receives little or no maintenance and is dominated by spontaneous vegetation – a cosmopolitan mix of species that grows and reproduces without human care or intent' (Del Tredici, 2010: 300) is the least studied of urban ecologies, which include different ages of vegetation, mosaics of successional stages, valuable structures and community ecology characteristics of edge habitat (Mathey and Rink, 2010). When buildings and land are abandoned, 'they offer a high number of niches which are, directly after abandonment, almost free of competition. Therefore, a large number of species is able to colonize these areas. Such early and intermediate states of succession have become very rare in the intensively used agricultural landscape' (Wittig, 2010: 44). In the UK wasteland or 'brownfield' areas are regarded as vital but overlooked habitats for UK wildlife, according to the charity Butterfly Conservation (Gill, 2012). These sites are home to unusual, hardy plants and their patches of bare ground provide warm microclimates that allow many rare insects to thrive. Furthermore, if left relatively undisturbed, wasteland provides 'a broad habitat mosaic and, consequently, opportunities to increase biodiversity' (Mathey and Rink, 2010: 409).

The course of succession as well as the composition of plant and animal species is influenced by climate, the intensity and type of former and current land use, neighbourhood effects, soil type and degree of soil permeability, and by the location and extent of urban wasteland. Succession in wasteland is usually recognised as moving through four stages (Mahey and Rink, 2010):

1. Young wasteland with pioneer vegetation (<3 years fallow period)
2. Older wasteland with persistent ruderal vegetation (pioneer plant species that colonise disturbed lands) (3-10 years fallow period)
3. Old wasteland with ruderal herbaceous vegetation (10-50 years fallow period)
4. Wasteland with spontaneous woodlands (> 50-year fallow period).

However, it is important to recognise that fallow wasteland does not have the same level of biodiversity throughout different successional stages. In those urban locations where forest represents the ecological climax, for example, it tends to be relatively species-poor compared to earlier stages (Wittig, 2010). In a study in Paris, Muratet et al (2007) found the largest number of plant species in vacant areas of medium age (4-13 years old).

In a study of Berlin, Zerbe et al (2003, 2004) found that the greatest variety of land use patterns and the highest number of species per area could be found in the transition zone between the city centre and the outskirts, where urban land use is associated with open spaces such as parks, urban forests and wastelands. The highest numbers of species were recorded in those habitats that were less intensively managed. However, land use patterns with moderate frequencies or intensities of disturbance positively affected habitat diversity, as well as overall species diversity. This therefore raises an important point that the species richness of wastefields can only be maintained by disrupting succession, which may require intervention (Wittig, 2010).

As Del Tredici (2010: 300, 302) points out, 'Perhaps the most obvious distinguishing aspect of urban environments is the ubiquitous physical disturbance associated with the construction and/or maintenance of their infrastructure. Such disturbances drastically alter existing soil and drainage characteristics, thereby changing the growing conditions for the associated biota.' The economic condition of the city may substantially influence the degree and nature of physical disturbance (Berger, 2006a). In economically vibrant cities, significant portions of the urban fabric are always being redeveloped. This tends to create a constantly shifting mosaic of opportunistic plant associations dominated by disturbance-tolerant, early successional species (Kowarik 2005; Del Tredici, 2010).

In more economically depressed cities, where a large percentage of the urban core and/or suburbs have been abandoned for significant periods of time, plant succession often proceeds without disturbance and achieves a more 'stable', multilayered structure than it does in more prosperous cities (Muratet et al, 2007; Del Tredici, 2010; Mathey and Rink, 2010). Using Leipzig as a case study, Mathey and Rink (2010) estimate that 5-7 per cent of the area in 'shrinking cities' is wasteland. This figure appears comparable to other research (Runfola and Hankins, 2009). Rink (2009) suggested that the amount and maturity of spontaneous vegetation that cities contain is inversely proportional to their economic prosperity.

'Enhancement of biodiversity in urban ecosystems can have a positive impact on the quality of life and education of urban dwellers and thus facilitate the preservation of biodiversity in natural ecosystems'

(Savard et al, 2000: 131). Wild ecologies can provide green space for play as well as moderate urban temperatures, especially important given concerns over climate change. However, 'many of the people who live in cities tend to interpret the presence of spontaneous urban vegetation in their neighborhood as a visible manifestation of dereliction and neglect, even though they may view the same plants growing in a suburban or rural context as "wildflowers"' (Del Tredici, 2010: 309). Even more pessimistically, Pyle (2003) suggests that urban populations are increasingly disconnected from the natural world, and are becoming evermore biophobic. Wilby and Perry (2006: 94) suggest that 'Clearly education and "reconnecting people with nature" are of prime importance if the biodiversity of urban habitats is to be protected.' Arguably this is even more important in the case of wastelands that already suffer an environmental image problem. For example, in June 2012 Butterfly Conservation and the insect magazine *Atropos* were encouraging people, where safe and legal access was possible, to explore their local quarries, disused railway lines, gravel pits and spoil tips in search of unusual moths. According to Richard Fox from Butterfly Conservation, many of the disturbed or even contaminated sites were under threat from redevelopment and 'bland landscaping schemes.... An old spoil tip [for example] would be terrible if you wanted to create a garden, but it's great for wildlife' (quoted in Gill, 2012).

Conclusion: valuing wasteland

The world's population is urbanising at a rapid rate: in 2010 51.6 per cent of the world's population was estimated to be living in urban areas, which compares to 36.6 per cent in 1970 and 29.4 per cent in 1950. It is estimated that by 2030 59.9 per cent of the global population will be living in urban areas and 67.2 per cent by 2050 (UN Department of Economic and Social Affairs, 2012). Such rates of urbanisation will lead to anthropogenic changes in land use, water quality (Shao et al, 2006), climate (Kalnay and Cai, 2003), air quality (Shao et al, 2006; Chan and Yao, 2008), connectivity of natural lands (Theobald et al, 1997), inputs of nutrients and toxic chemicals (Groffman et al, 2004; Hatt et al, 2004), and biological diversity (Blair, 1996; Wang et al, 2001; Secretariat of the Convention on Biological Diversity, 2010). Nevertheless, the promotion of urban biodiversity can help counter many of these changes and increase the provision of environmental services within the city.

Urban biodiversity also serves important functions relating to mitigation and adaptation to climate change. Vegetation helps reduce the urban heat island effect, thereby 'cooling' cities. The annual mean temperatures of large urban areas can be up to 3°C warmer than the surrounding non-urban areas, and on extreme occasions the temperature difference between the city and the surrounding countryside can even be as high as 12°C (Sieghardt et al, 2005). Vegetation also acts as carbon storage. In a study of the amount of vegetation across Leicester, a British city with a population of about 300,000 people, it was estimated that 231,000 tonnes of carbon, equivalent to 3.16kg m^2, was locked away in the city's vegetation – most of which was stored by trees (Davies et al, 2011). The assessment included domestic gardens, public spaces, road verges and derelict industrial land.

The development of land recycling is characterised by a reciprocal process in comparison to the system of waste recycling, where useless matter is turned into useful matter (Erz, 1992; Strasser, 1992). Thompson's (1979) rubbish theory, which claims that objects move both into and out of the category of rubbish, can be applied to the case of wasteland. It can also be applied to Strasser's (1992: 8) observation that 'objects ... no longer desired by some' are (now) 'desirable to others', when we regard the increasing desire of a growing part of industrial society for wasteland as a conservation asset. Yet at the same time that there is encouragement for recognition of the ecological values of wasteland, there are counter-arguments to allowing the ecological succession of wasteland, not so much for their aesthetic qualities, but because of the extent that derelict land reveals environmental injustice (see also Chapter Eleven). As Lynch (1990a: 115) observed, 'Wastes are traditionally dumped at the edges of settlement – in areas where the powerless live, where land claims are weak, and where controls are soft.'

Runfola and Hankins' (2009) study of urban dereliction in Atlantic City surveyed the distribution of urban neglect and the presence (or absence) of resident activism in both high- and low-dereliction areas. The study indicated that some residents in high-dereliction areas, while acutely aware of dereliction and actively involved in neighbourhood and community organisations, had been unsuccessful in pressuring city government agencies to enforce code violations and to maintain the physical infrastructure. 'Residents in mostly minority, low-income, medium- or high-dereliction areas, while active in a variety of civic groups, find themselves with inadequate response from the city in addressing environmental concerns, ranging from abandoned houses to trash collection' (Runfola and Hankins, 2009: 362). This is significant as it only served to reinforce the uneven geographies of urban neglect. Yet the maintenance of urban biodiversity should not come at the cost of neighbourhood neglect.

Wastelands, as with waste (O'Connell, 2011), constitute a landscape of fear for some. The core problem for the development and maintenance of urban ecologies is that 'wastelands are often perceived by residents as a sign of decay and decline and the wild spontaneous nature often regarded as a sign that the city is not being run well' (Dettmar, 2005: 408). Lynch (1972: 192) also had similar concerns, suggesting that 'wasteland creates a disturbing image of death and decay. Yet economic growth and exterior change will often require gradual emigration and progressive abandonment.' Wasteland, like much waste in the city (see Chapters One and Three), is therefore regarded as an artefact of economic growth and change. Yet in the same way that narratives of 'natural' wilderness have changed, so have understandings of wasteland in the city. 'The labeling of something as waste must always ask: waste for whom?' (Lynch 1990a: 148). As Hough (2004: 6) observed, 'If we make the not unreasonable assumption that diversity is ecologically and socially necessary to the health and quality of urban life, then we must question the values that determine the image of nature in cities.'

Dunnett et al (2002) found that the quality and maintenance of green spaces was likely to be viewed by local residents as one of the main indicators of neighbourhood quality. However, in terms of promoting urban biodiversity, there needs to be a shift in many Western cities in the landscape ideal being 'lawn' to something that is more naturalistic, if not indigenous. Yet urban ecosystem services are not just provided by native species. In the same way that ecologists have only recently recognised that a measurable degree of ecological functionality can be achieved with a cosmopolitan assemblage of species (Hobbs et al, 2009), so city residents also need to reassess the environmental and aesthetic properties of wasteland environments. Wastelands in cities is anything but: they have high ecological values, contribute substantially to urban ecosystem services, reducing the ecological footprint of the city, and also fulfil understandings of sustainable landscapes in the sense that they are (1) adapted to their site; (2) require minimal maintenance; (3) are ecologically and socially functional; and (4) are cost-effective (Kühn, 2006; Del Tredici, 2010). In addition, some wasteland areas may be suitable for use as short- and long-term community gardens, or for development for urban agriculture (Smit and Nasr, 1992). Although these are usually non-native plantings, they still provide significant ecosystem and community services, and can also contribute to the maintenance of urban invertebrate populations, especially insects (Hough, 2004).

Changing understandings and narratives of wastelands means realising that 'Cities are not static objects, but active arenas marked by continuous energy flows and transformations of which landscapes and buildings and other hard parts are not permanent structures but transitional manifestations' (Berger, 2006b: 203). As Berger went on to note, 'the challenge for designers is thus not to achieve *drossless* urbanization but to integrate inevitable dross into a more flexible aesthetic and design strategies' (Berger 2006b: 203, emphasis in original). So-called reclamation and regeneration projects therefore need to consider the environmental value of the spontaneous ecologies of wasteland and to engage in development practices that work with such nature. Indeed, as Del Tredici (2010: 310) suggests, 'design approaches which integrate the ecological functionality, aesthetic appearance, and recreational potential of spontaneous urban woodlands [and other wasteland vegetation] are more likely to succeed than those which focus on ecology alone.' This means that (1) people are an integral part of the urban habitat and that their preferences need to be part of the management plans; (2) careful manipulation of natural successional processes can enhance the aesthetic qualities of urban environments; and (3) the insertion of well-designed landscape features, such as pathways, facilitates their use by people, thereby generating political support for their preservation (Del Tredici, 2010: 310; cf Kowarik, 2005). In some cases this will mean encouraging the development of wild urban ecologies; in others this may mean encouraging the development of urban agricultural and community-based vegetable gardens, the two approaches being compatible in many cases. Most importantly, the core narrative that needs to be adopted is that wasteland is not a waste.

References

Barr, J. (1969) *Derelict Britain*, Harmondsworth: Penguin Books.

Berger, A. (2006a) 'Drosscape in the landscape', in C. Waldheim (ed) *The urbanism reader*, Princeton, NJ: Princeton University Press, pp 197-217.

Berger, A. (2006b) *Drosscape: Wasting land in urban America*, New York: Princeton Architectural Press.

Berger, A. (ed) (2008) *Designing the reclaimed landscape*, New York: Routledge.

Blair, R.B. (1996) 'Land use and avian species diversity along an urban gradient', *Ecological Applications*, vol 6, pp 506-19.

Blaustein, J. (2011) *Urban media lab: Waste*, New York: The New School University, Department of Media Studies and Film.

Boeri, S. (1993) 'New nameless spaces', *Casabella*, vol 57, no 597/598, pp 74-76, 123-4.

Boffet, A. and Rocca Serra, S. (2001) 'Identification of spatial structures within urban blocks for town characterisation', in *Proceedings of the 20th International Cartographic Conference*, Beijing, China.

Bowman, A.O. and Pagano, M.A. (2000) 'Transforming America's cities: Policies and conditions of vacant land', *Urban Affairs Review*, vol 35, no 4, pp 559-81.

Chan, C.K. and Yao, X. (2008) 'Air pollution in mega cities in China', *Atmospheric Environment*, vol 42, no 1, pp 1-42.

Cheung, W.-T.P. (2000) 'Reinterpretation and interaction, the neglected urban landscape', Thesis, Master's in Landscape Architecture, Department of Landscape Architecture, University of Manitoba.

Clapp, J.A. (2005) '"Are you talking to me?" – New York and the cinema of urban alienation', *Visual Anthropology*, vol 18, no 1, pp 1-18.

Davies, Z.G., Edmondson, J.L., Heinemeyer, A., Leake, J.R. and Gaston, K.J. (2011) 'Mapping an urban ecosystem service: quantifying above-ground carbon storage at a city-wide scale', *Journal of Applied Ecology*, vol 48, no 5, pp 1125-34.

Dehaene, M. and de Cauter, L. (eds) (2008) *Heterotopia and the city: Public space in a postcivil society*, London: Routledge.

de Sola-Morales, R.I. (1995) 'Terrain vague', in C.C. Davidson (ed) *Anyplace*, London: The MIT Press, pp 119-23.

Del Tredici, P. (2010) 'Spontaneous urban vegetation: Reflections of change in a globalized world', *Nature and Culture*, vol 5, no 3, pp 299-315.

Dettmar, J. (2005) 'Forests for shrinking cities? The project "Industrial Forests in the Ruhr"', in I. Kowarik and S. Körner (eds) *Wild urban woodlands*, Berlin: Springer-Verlag, pp 263-76.

Doron, G. (2000) 'The dead zone and the architecture of transgression', *CITY, Analysis of Urban Trends, Culture, Theory, Policy, Action*, vol 4, no 2, pp 247-64.

Doron, G. (2008) '… those marvellous empty zones at the edge of cities', in M. Dehaene and L. de Cauter (eds) *Heterotopia and the city: Public space in a postcivil society*, London: Routledge, pp 203-14.

Dunnett, N., Swanwick, C. and Woolley, H. (2002) *Improving urban parks, play areas and green spaces*, London: Department for Transport, Local Government and the Regions.

Edensor, T. (2005) *Industrial ruins*, New York: Berg.

Endsjø, D.O. (2000) 'To lock up Eleusis: A question of liminal space', *Numen*, vol 47, no 4, 351-86.

Erz, W. (1992) 'Wasteland: Land for conservation', in *Waste and want. The other side of consumption, Susan Strasser with comments by Gunther Barth and Wolfgang Erz*, Annual Lecture Series No 5, German Historical Institute, Washington, DC, Providence, RI: Berg, pp 29-34.

Eshel, A. (2003) 'Cosmopolitanism and searching for the sacred space in Jewish literature', *Jewish Social Studies, New Series*, vol 9, no 3, pp 121-38.

Farley, P. and Roberts, M.S. (2011) *Edgelands: Journeys into England's true wilderness*, London: Jonathan Cape.

Foucault, M. (1998) 'Different spaces' (translated by M. Hurley), in J.D. Faubion (ed) *Aesthetics, method, and epistemology: Essential works of Foucault, Volume 2*, London: Penguin, pp 175-85.

Funk, R.W. (1959) 'The wilderness', *Journal of Biblical Literature*, vol 78, pp 205-14.

Gill, V. (2012) 'Waste land or "brownfield" sites are vital for wildlife', BBC Nature, 21 June (www.bbc.co.uk/nature/18513022).

Godefroid, S. and Koedam, N. (2007) 'Urban plant species are highly driven by density and function of built-up areas', *Landscape Ecology*, vol 22, pp 1227-39.

Greenberg, M. and Schneider, D. (1996) *Environmentally devastated neighborhoods: Perceptions, policies, and realities*, New Brunswick, NJ: Rutgers University Press.

Grimm, D. and Dosch, F. (2010) 'Brownfield management in Germany: A sustainable issue', *Journal of Urban Regeneration and Renewal*, vol 3, no 3, pp 246-62.

Groffman, P.M., Law, N.L., Belt, K.T., Band, L.E. and Fisher, G.T. (2004) 'Nitrogen fluxes and retention in urban watershed ecosystems', *Ecosystems*, vol 7, pp 393-403.

Guttenberg, A.Z. (1978) 'City encounter and "desert" encounter: two sources of American regional planning thought', *Journal of the American Institute of Planners*, vol 44, no 4, pp 399-411.

Haase, D. (2008) 'Urban ecology of shrinking cities: An unrecognized opportunity?', *Nature and Culture*, vol 3, no 1, pp 1-8.

Haid, C. (2011) 'Landscapes of wilderness – Heterotopias of the post-industrial city', Paper presented at 'Framing the city', Manchester: Royal Northern College of Music.

Hall, C.M. (1989) 'The worthless lands hypothesis and Australia's national parks and reserves', in K. Frawley and N. Semple (eds) *Australia's ever changing forests*, Canberra: Department of Geography Monograph Series, Australian Defence Force Academy, pp 441-56.

Hall, C.M. (1992) *From wasteland to world heritage: Conserving Australia's wilderness*, Melbourne: Melbourne University Press.

Hall, C.M. and Frost, W. (2009) 'National parks and the "worthless lands hypothesis" revisited', in W. Frost and C.M. Hall (eds) *Tourism and national parks: International perspectives on development, histories and change*, London: Routledge, pp 45-62.

Hatt, B.E., Fletcher, T.D., Walsh, C.J. and Taylor, S.L. (2004) 'The influence of urban density and drainage infrastructure on the concentrations and loads of pollutants in small streams', *Environmental Management*, vol 34, pp 112-24.

Hobbs, R.J., Higgs, E. and Harris, J.A. (2009) 'Novel ecosystems: Implications for conservation and restoration', *Trends in Ecology and Evolution*, vol 24, no 11, pp 599-605.

Hormigo, P. and Morita, T. (2004) 'Urban *gapscapes*: Problems and opportunities in urban design analysis of *gapspaces* originated by elevated railways', *Journal of Asian Architecture and Building Engineering*, vol 3, no 1, pp 181-8.

Hough, M. (2004) *Cities and natural processes: A basis for sustainability* (2nd edn), New York: Routledge.

Jackson, S. (1997) 'A disturbing story: The fiction of rationality in land use planning in Aboriginal Australia', *Australian Planner*, vol 34, no 3, pp 221-6.

Jakle, J.A. and Wilson, D. (1992) *Derelict landscapes: The wasting of America's built environment*, Savage, MD: Rowman & Littlefield Publishers.

Johnson, P. (2006) 'Unravelling Foucault's different spaces', *History of the Human Sciences*, vol 19, no 4, pp 75-90.

Kalnay, E. and Cai, M. (2003) 'Impact of urbanization and land-use change on climate', *Nature*, vol 423, pp 528-31.

Kennedy, G. (2007) *An ontology of trash: The disposable and its problematic nature*, Albany, NY: State University of New York Press.

Klotz, S. (1990) 'Species/area and species/inhabitants relations in European cities', in H. Sukopp, S. Hejný and I. Kowarik (eds) *Urban ecology*, The Hague: SPB Academic Publishing, pp 99-104.

Kowarik, I. (2005) 'Wild urban woodlands: Toward a conceptual framework', in I. Kowarik and S. Körner (eds) *Wild urban woodlands*, Berlin: Springer, pp 1-32.

Kühn, N. (2006) 'Intentions for the unintentional spontaneous vegetation as the basis for innovative planting design in urban areas', *Journal of Landscape Architecture*, vol 1, no 2, pp 46-53.

Lerup, L. (2006) *After the city*, Cambridge, MA: The MIT Press.

Lynch, K. (1972) *What time is this place?*, Cambridge, MA: The MIT Press.

Lynch, K. (1990a) *Wasting away* (edited by M. Southworth), San Francisco, CA: Sierra Club Books.

Lynch, K. (1990b) 'The waste of place', *Places: Forum of Design for the Public Realm*, vol 6, no 2, pp 10-23.

Mathey, J. and Rink, D. (2010) 'Urban wasteland – a change for biodiversity in cities? Ecological aspects, social perceptions and acceptance of wilderness by residents', in N. Müller, P. Werner and J.G. Kelcey (eds) *Urban biodiversity and design*, Oxford: Wiley-Blackwell, pp 406-24.

Müller, N., Werner, P. and Kelcey, J.G. (eds) (2010) *Urban biodiversity and design*, Oxford: Wiley-Blackwell.

Muratet, A., Machon, N., Jiguet, F., Moret, J. and Porcher, E. (2007) 'The role of urban structures in the distribution of wasteland flora in the greater Paris area, France', *Ecosystems*, vol 19, no 4, pp 661-71.

Nash, R. (1982) *Wilderness and the American mind* (3rd edn), New Haven, CT: Yale University Press.

O'Connell, E. (2011) 'Overcoming the fear of waste', *Waste Management*, vol 31, no 11, pp 2201-2.

Oxenham, J.R. (1966) *Reclaiming derelict land*, London: Faber & Faber.

Puth, L.M. and Burns, C.E. (2009) 'New York's nature: a review of the status and trends in species richness across the metropolitan region', *Diversity and Distributions*, vol 15, pp 12-21.

Pyle, R.M. (2003) 'Nature matrix: reconnecting people and nature', *Oryx*, vol 37, pp 206-14.

Pysek, P. (1989) 'On the richness of central European urban flora', *Preslia*, vol 61, pp 329-34.

Pysek, P. (1993) 'Factors affecting the diversity of flora and vegetation in central European settlements', *Vegetatio*, vol 106, pp 89-100.

Ramson, W. (1991) 'Wasteland to wilderness: changing perceptions of the environment', in D.J. Mulvaney (ed) *The humanities and the Australian environment*, Canberra: Australian Academy of the Humanities, pp 5-19.

Rink, D. (2009) 'Wilderness: The nature of urban shrinkage? The debate on urban restructuring and restoration in eastern Germany', *Nature and Culture*, vol 4, no 3, pp 275-92.

Runfola, D.M. and Hankins, K.M. (2009) 'Urban dereliction as environmental injustice', *ACME: An International E-Journal for Critical Geographies*, vol 9, no 3, pp 345-67.

Runte, A. (1972) 'Yellowstone: it's useless, so why not a park', *National Parks and Conservation Magazine*, vol 46, March, pp 4-7.

Runte, A. (1973) '"Worthless" lands – our national parks: the enigmatic past and uncertain future of America's scenic wonderlands', *American West*, vol 10, May, pp 4-11.

Savard, J.P.L., Clergeau, P. and Mennechez, G. (2000) 'Biodiversity concepts and urban ecosystems', *Landscape and Urban Planning*, vol 48, pp 131-42.

Secretariat of the Convention on Biological Diversity (2010) *Global biodiversity outlook 3*, Montreal: Secretariat of the Convention on Biological Diversity.

Shao, M., Tang, X.Y., Zhang, Y.H. and Li, W.J. (2006) 'City clusters in China: air and surface water pollution', *Frontiers in Ecology and the Environment*, vol 4, no 7, pp 353-61.

Sieghardt, M., Mursch-Radlgruber, E., Paoletti, E., Couenberg, E., Dimitrakopoulus, A., Rego, F., Hatzistathis, A. and Randrup, T.B. (2005) 'The abiotic environment: impact of urban growing conditions on urban vegetation', in C.C. Konijnendijk, K. Nilsson, T.B. Randrup, and J. Schipperijn (eds) *Urban forests and trees*, Berlin: Springer, pp 281-323.

Southworth, M. (2001) *Wastelands in the evolving metropolis*, IURD Working Paper 2001-01, Berkeley, CA: Institute of Urban and Regional Development, University of California.

Smit, J. and Nasr, J. (1992) 'Urban agriculture for sustainable cities: using wastes and idle land and water bodies as resources', *Environment and Urbanization*, vol 4, no 2, pp 141-52.

Strasser, S. (1992) 'Waste and want: The other side of consumption', in *Waste and want. The other side of consumption, Susan Strasser with comments by Gunther Barth and Wolfgang Erz*, Annual Lecture Series No 5, German Historical Institute, Washington, DC, Providence, RI: Berg, pp 5-21.

Strom, A.A. (1979) 'Impressions of a developing conservation ethic, 1870-1930', *Parks and Wildlife*, vol 2, nos 3-4, pp 45-53.

Theobald, D.M., Miller, J.R. and Hobbs, N.T. (1997) 'Estimating the cumulative effects of development on wildlife habitat', *Landscape and Urban Planning*, vol 39, pp 25-36.

Thompson, M. (1979) *Rubbish theory: The creation and destruction of value*, Oxford: Oxford University Press.

Tuan, Y.-F. (1974) *Topophilia: A study of environmental perception, attitudes, and values*, Englewood Cliffs, NJ: Prentice-Hall.

UN (United Nations) Department of Economic and Social Affairs, Population Division (2012) *World urbanization prospects: The 2011 revision*, CD-ROM edition, Data in digital form (POP/ DB/WUP/ Rev.2011), New York: UN Department of Economic and Social Affairs, Population Division, Population Estimates and Projects Section.

Walters, S.M. (1970) 'The next twenty years', in I. Perring (ed), *The flora of a changing Britain*, Hampton: Botanical Society of the British Isles & Classey, pp 136-41.

Wang, L.Z., Lyons, J. and Kanehl, P. (2001) 'Impacts of urbanization on stream habitat and fish across multiple spatial scales', *Environmental Management*, vol 28, pp 255-66.

Wilby, R.L. and Perry, G.L.W. (2006) 'Climate change, biodiversity and the urban environment: a critical review based on London, UK', *Progress in Physical Geography*, vol 30, no 1, pp 73-98.

Wittig, R. (2010) 'Biodiversity of urban-industrial areas and its evaluation – a critical review', in N. Müller, P. Werner and J.G. Kelcey (eds) *Urban biodiversity and design*, Oxford: Wiley-Blackwell, pp 37-55.

Woods, L. (2000) 'No-man's land', in A. Read (ed) *Architecturally speaking: Practices of art, architecture and the everyday*, London: Routledge, pp 199-210.

Zerbe, S., Maurer, U., Schmitz, S. and Sukopp, H. (2003) 'Biodiversity in Berlin and its potential for nature conservation', *Landscape and Urban Planning*, vol 62, no 3, pp 139-48.

Zerbe, S., Maurer, U., Peschel, T., Schmitz, S. and Sukopp, H. (2004) 'Diversity of flora and vegetation in European cities as a potential for nature conservation in urban-industrial areas – with examples from Berlin and Potsdam (Germany)', in W.W. Shaw, L.K. Harris and L. Vandruff (eds) *Proceedings of the 4th International Urban Wildlife Symposium*, Tuscon, AZ: School of Natural Resources, College of Agriculture and Life Sciences, University of Arizona, pp 35-49.

Zeveloff, S.I., Vause, L.M. and McVaugh, W.H. (eds) *Wilderness tapestry: An eclectic approach to preservation*, Reno, NV: University of Nevada Press.

THREE

The function of waste urban infrastructures as heterotopias of the city: narratives from Gothenburg and Managua

María José Zapata Campos

Introduction

This chapter uses the notion of heterotopia (Foucault, 1986) to rethink the functions and meanings of waste urban infrastructures, based on narratives of waste from the cities of Managua in Nicaragua and Gothenburg in Sweden. A heterotopia is a physical representation of a utopia, or a parallel space that contains undesirable bodies to make a real utopian space possible, such as a prison or a cemetery. Foucault divides all spaces into ordinary and extraordinary. The extraordinary are divided into utopias, or unreal places, and heterotopias, which are real:

> There are also, probably in every culture, in every civilization, real places – places that do exist and that are formed in the very founding of society – which are something like counter-sites, a kind of effectively enacted utopia in which the real sites, all the other real sites that can be found within the culture, are simultaneously represented, contested, and inverted. Places of this kind are outside of all places, even though it may be possible to indicate their location in reality. (Foucault 1986: 24)

Although Foucault did not mention them as such, waste urban infrastructures such as landfill sites or incinerators are heterotopic places. Waste urban infrastructures constitute 'the other city' where citizens cast out their wasted things. Waste urban infrastructures hold as heterotopias relevant roles and functions, which vary between different societies: 'A society, as its history unfolds can make an existing heterotopia function in a very different fashion; for each heterotopia has a precise and determined function within a society and the same heterotopia can, according to the synchrony of the culture in which it occurs, have one function or another' (Foucault 1986: 25).

The analysis of the functions of waste urban infrastructures presented in this chapter is based on the narratives collected from two ordinary cities: Managua in Nicaragua and Gothenburg in Sweden (Amin and Graham, 1997; Graham and Marvin, 2001; Robinson, 2006, 2011). To compare a wealthy city in the global North such as Gothenburg, in one of the wealthiest countries in the world, with Managua, the capital of Nicaragua, the second poorest country of the Americas, might appear methodologically and ontologically inappropriate. However, cities are best understood as ordinary rather than labelling them as Western, third world, developed, developing or global (Robinson, 2006: 1). This chapter argues that it is important for cities in wealthy societies 'to be open to learning from the experiences of poor cities' (Robinson, 2006: 141), especially when the differences between one or the other are lessening (Graham and Thrift, 2007).

Following the ethnographic work of Star (1999) regarding the understanding of infrastructures, this chapter focuses on the reading and 'unfreezing of waste infrastructures' and their taken-for-granted work. In order to do that it performs what Bowker (Bowker and Star, 1989) called an 'infrastructural inversion'. The chapter is based on observations conducted in waste infrastructures in the two cities: the city dump of Managua, La Chureca and some of its spontaneous settlements, and the Sävenäs waste incinerator in Gothenburg. Photographs, field notes with observations, personal interviews and document analysis collected as part of two waste research programmes constitute the main source of data.

The chapter next presents the narratives of waste collected in the cities of Managua and Gothenburg. It then analyses the functions of waste urban infrastructures based on these narratives through the notion of heterotopias. The chapter concludes with a discussion about how to invert waste infrastructures and make visible their 'taken-for-granted' work.

Narratives of waste from Managua

Managua is the capital city of Nicaragua in Central America. Almost 1.5 out of the six million inhabitants in the country live in the city, with almost half of the national population concentrated in the metropolitan region. As in many Latin American cities, rural migration has resulted in rapid and unplanned over-urbanisation. As a consequence, more than one third of Managua consists of spontaneous settlements (Parés Barberena, 2006), and one of the basic urban services missing in these spontaneous settlements is waste collection.

The provision of the household waste management service in Managua has become a hybrid between the formal collection system provided by the municipality, and informal services provided by scavengers, waste collector cooperatives and other informal micro-enterprises (see Chapter Five). The waste municipal service is currently limited to the disposal of waste at La Chureca, the municipal rubbish dump. At La Chureca, hospital, electronic and hazardous waste are all disposed of together, and the dump lacked a sanitary landfill until 2012. As a consequence, the permanent flow of leachate leaking from the landfill has been contaminating the nearby Lake Xolotlán for decades. Similarly, the spontaneous combustion of the waste accumulated for decades is heavily contaminating the nearby neighbourhood of Acahualinca and the city of Managua. With more than 2,000 scavengers working daily at La Chureca to recover valuable materials from the rubbish, the inhuman conditions in which they are working has resulted in a number of diseases, labour accidents and infections (Grigsby, 2008).

In the city of Managua, the lack of accessibility to the spontaneous settlements, together with the shortage of municipal resources, means that an important number of *barrios* (neighbourhoods) remain out of the official waste collection service. In the city districts six and seven it was estimated that 33 per cent of households were not attended at all by the municipal waste collection service (UNDP, 2009) and, if they were, the service was irregular and insufficient. Some of the families visited in the Barrios Betancourt and Olof Palme settlements only had access to this service once or twice a month. So, the local population has developed a number of coping strategies in order to access basic urban infrastructures illegally, such as water, electricity and/or waste removal. Labouring children, scavengers and other groups collect household waste, sorting out what is recyclable and sellable, and dumping the rest in illegal dumps. As a result, waste is present and visible everywhere in the *barrios*; streets, roadside ditches, gutters, drains, riverbanks or barrels are flooded with waste. And a minority of organised groups have started collecting recyclables and household waste using traditional transport means, such as bicycles or horses, to provide a regular household waste collection service to the neighbours of some of these *barrios*.

Both the formal and informal household waste collection system in Managua is carried out with the sound of a bell hanging from the waste municipal trucks, or a whistle used by the cart men (Zapata Campos and Zapata, 2013). In this way they announce to the residents that the waste collection service is approaching their homes. Residents then go out from their houses and dispose of their waste directly to the waste collectors without human or even non-human intermediaries (see Figure 3.1). Only a reusable bag separates the waste householder from the waste collector. Waste becomes visible to the eyes of everybody when the collectors empty the bags into the carts or the trucks, exposing the contents and returning the bag to the householder to be reused for the next service. The waste flow exits the privacy of the home to enter the public domain; from this moment waste becomes a public responsibility. The exchange of waste from the private to the public sphere is evident, direct, and occurs with more transparent intermediating technologies, accountabilities or procedures. In the case of the official municipal waste service, a municipal tax, paid irregularly to the municipal department, mediates this exchange, while the service provided by the cart men is paid at the very moment the waste is collected.

Figure 3.1: Waste collection in Managua's informal settlements

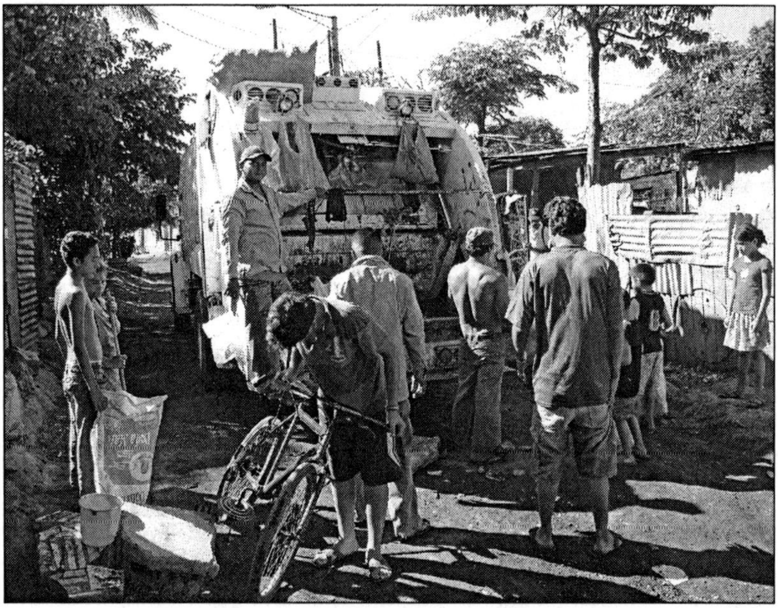

Narratives of waste from Gothenburg

Approximately 920,000 people live in the Gothenburg region. Renova AB, the municipal company owned by the 11 municipalities in this region, has been in charge of the handling of household waste and its collection in most of the municipalities since 1972. The key waste handling process is incineration with energy recovery in the public-owned incineration plant, Sävenäs. The incinerated waste creates energy, which is used for heating and electricity. The plant produces 5 per cent of the electricity and 30 per cent of the district heating consumed in the region (Renova, 2011a, 2011b). The way Renova, and other waste handling companies in Sweden, process waste is based on the European Union (EU) waste hierarchy: reducing waste, reusing materials, recovering materials through recycling, recovering energy and, as the last alternative, landfilling. The EU Waste Framework Directive (2008/98/EC) encourages the elimination of landfilling and, as a last resort, supports waste incineration activities. The new laws, however, give priority to waste prevention and encourage reuse and recovery of waste, demanding a change of focus from recycling and incineration (Swedish Environmental Agency, 2011).

In the inner city of Gothenburg is Nordostpassagen, a social housing project constructed at the end of the 1960s, which has been renewed and revalued due to its central location. The houses are equipped with a vacuum waste collection system. Residents just need to carry their rubbish bags a few metres, open the circular door in the wall and throw it into the pipe whenever necessary (see Figure 3.2). The rubbish bag just disappears. This is one of the technological devices that make waste most invisible. As the company responsible for its installation and maintenance puts it, the vacuum waste collection system is 'the invisible solution for environmentally sustainable waste handling' (Envac, 2012). This vacuum collection system does not allow for the disposal of all rubbish, however. The residents association states rules about what can and cannot be disposed of in the pipe. Similarly, there are municipal laws, based on national and European directives, that regulate what is waste, what can be collected and not, where, when and how. Despite this, the residents, hidden by the anonymity provided by the privacy of the waste vacuum pipe or the waste room, sometimes break these rules, abandoning the most bizarre objects. Once the waste bag is thrown into the pipe it goes to the basement, and it is stored there until one of Renova's trucks comes to collect it. Access to the basement waste room is extremely restricted: only Renova's technical officers can enter. Mixed waste is then transported in the Renova waste trucks to the Sävenäs incinerator, where it becomes fuel to be transformed into clean energy. When the trucks dispose of the waste at the incinerator, it is, again, visible, although only partially, since the mountain of waste

Figure 3.2: Waste vacuum chute, Nordostpassagen

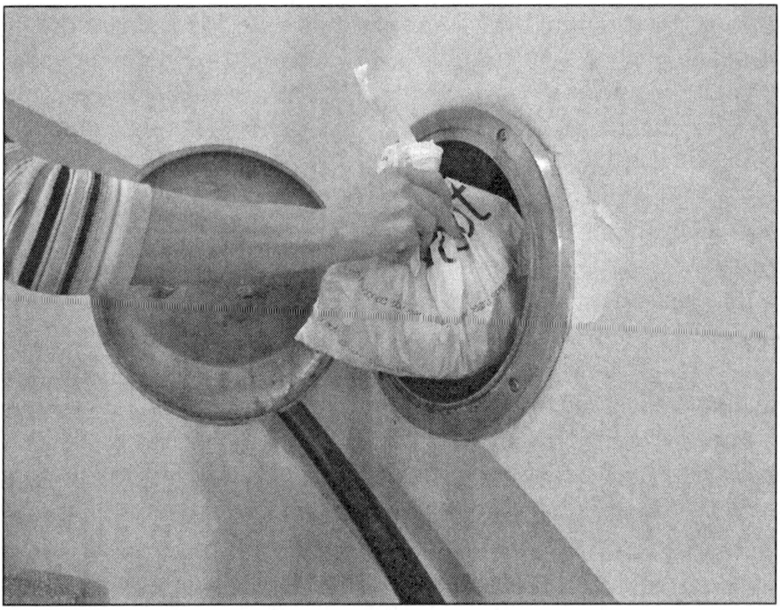

at the bottom of the bunker is made up of a mix of heterogeneous materials and fluids.

Waste incinerators such as Sävenäs are presented in Renova's discourse as a 'dioxin sink', contributing to the reduction of the impacts of climate change on cities:

> 'Some of us say that waste incineration is a low point of dioxins ... it is a place where we destroy more dioxides than are formed. There are dioxins in society, we are taking them to the incineration plants and dioxins are destroyed by the heat in the incineration process. Actually less emissions come out from the chimney than what it came in with waste. The question is that Sävenäs is a dioxin sink in society.' (Renova's officer during one lecture at Sävenäs)

> When biological waste is deposited in landfills and breaks down, methane – which is a particularly damaging greenhouse gas – is formed. At the waste-to-energy plant in Sävenäs, instead we transform that waste into energy. This helps to reduce pollution in our communities as well. By burning the waste and cleaning the emissions to the air and water effectively, we are taking environmentally damaging

> substances out of circulation in the natural environment. (Renova, 2012: 5)

After combustion, around 20 per cent by weight and 5-10 per cent by volume of the waste remains as slag. What cannot be recycled is transported to landfills such as Tagene. 'The last resort: terminal storage in landfills of waste that cannot be recycled. Renova's two landfills were constructed to very strict environmental requirements to be safe for a long time into the future. These are modern landfills, where waste is deposited pending new recycling methods' (Renova, 2012: 6). Slag is temporarily disposed of into a kind of limbo, pending the development of new technological solutions that might salvage or recover materials or energy from it.

Functions of waste urban infrastructures as heterotopias of the city

In this section the functions of waste urban infrastructures are analysed through the notion of heterotopias and based on the narratives of waste presented above. First, we discuss how waste infrastructures function as a mirror of society, and how they enable us to understand the society they reflect. Then, we look at how waste infrastructures make possible the utopia of a well-functioning city, by isolating and hiding waste for some parts of our societies and in some places in our cities. Finally, we discuss the implications of these findings for a sustainable urban development and social and environmental justice in the city.

Waste infrastructures as a mirror of society

While the utopia of the city is an unreal space representing the image of a perfectly functioning city, heterotopia of the city are real places, such as waste infrastructures, that enact the utopic city. Foucault uses the metaphor of the mirror to explain the relationship between utopias and heterotopias:

> The mirror is, after all, a utopia, since it is a placeless place. In the mirror, I see myself there where I am not, in an unreal, virtual space that opens up behind the surface; I am over there, there where I am not, a sort of shadow that gives my own visibility to myself, that enables me to see myself there where I am absent: such is the utopia of the mirror(…). The mirror (also) functions as a heterotopia in this respect: it

> makes this place that I occupy at the moment when I look at myself in the glass at once absolutely real, connected with all the space that surrounds it. (Foucault 1986: 24)

Accordingly, waste urban infrastructures become the artefact (the mirror itself, the heterotopia) that makes it possible to understand what a society resembles by providing its reflection.

Some waste infrastructures provide a historical reflection of the cities and the societies in which they are embedded. 'Heterotopias are most often linked to slices in time' (Foucault, 1986: 26); they are breaks in the traditional understanding of time, called by Foucault heterochronies, or 'other times'. Landfill sites or incinerator bunkers, as with cemeteries or museums, are highly heterotopic places since they begin with 'this strange heterochrony, the loss of (social and physical) life' of things, 'and with this quasi-eternity in which her permanent lot is dissolution and disappearance' (Foucault, 1986: 26). Although most waste urban infrastructures are, nowadays, transitory places, some waste infrastructures such as landfill sites retain the property of accumulating time. Indeed, it is from the discards of former civilisations that archeologists have reconstructed most of what we know about the past (Rathje and Murphy, 1991), meaning that sealed and reconverted sanitary landfill sites will probably become the archeological sites of future researchers.

It is through the study of today's society's rubbish that 'garbology' was born as part of the archeology of the present and its outcasts. The rationale is that the understanding of the consumption patterns in society can be better, and more trustfully, understood by researching its rubbish than by asking consumers about their behaviour (Rathje and Murphy, 1991). This is because waste infrastructures also reflect the society in which they are embedded. Waste urban infrastructures are places connected with all the sites of the city simultaneously, and containing in them somehow part of the other real sites. As heterotopic places, waste infrastructures collect together in 'a single real place, several sites that [would be] in themselves incompatible' (Foucault, 1986: 25). In the ordinary city, wealthy and poor city dwellers, industry and households, all dispose of their 'dead' objects in these infrastructures. City dumps such as La Chureca in Managua fully fit this description where meat, industrial waste, old newspapers, the dead bodies of animals or even humans eventually lay side by side (see Figure 3.3). Even in highly modern European Nordic cities such as Gothenburg, food, books and bicycles lay together in the bunker of the waste incinerator.

Figure 3.3: La Chureca rubbish dump, Managua

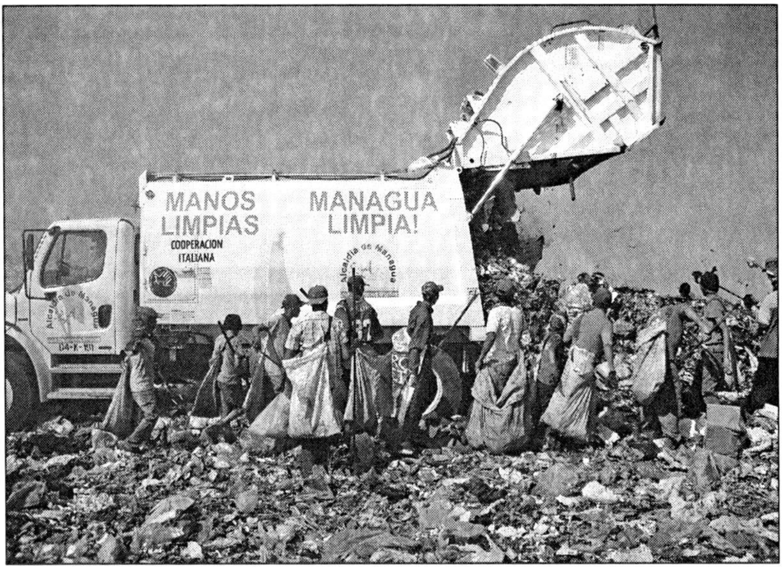

Journalists have also efficiently used garbology as a research method, exploring people's private lives. For example, as a result of research on the origin of the glass bottles and metal cans dumped and collected by the Swedish National Association of Glass Recyclers, the Gothenburg Press (2011) reported that the illegal imported alcohol trade in Sweden was much larger than what official reports had estimated. In the narratives collected from Gothenburg, one of the municipal waste managers mentioned how, "We [the waste incineration infrastructure] are the mirror of society." The Swedish Environmental Protection Agency has also asked the managers of the waste incineration facilities to investigate how many pollutants are present in society by analysing its waste. "The environmental agency of Sweden considers us as a mirror of the society so they want to know how many pollutants are in waste" (Renova's officer during one lecture at Sävenäs).

Given that waste urban infrastructures are a mirror of society, the flow of waste, its composition and volume will vary according to sociotechnological changes and place context. In Managua 70 per cent of its waste was organic due to the lower levels of consumption, industrialisation and economic development. In contrast, in Gothenburg other types of waste, such as electronic waste, is increasing dramatically year on year, and is being exported to 'third world' countries for material disassemby in economies with lower labour costs and probably less restrictive working and environmental conditions. During one of the guided tours in Sävenäs, we learned how, although 'waste does not take a vacation', industrial and household waste decreases considerably during the summer; one more example of how waste infrastructures reflect the society in which they are embedded.

Heterotopic waste urban infrastructures and the utopia of the well-functioning city

Waste urban infrastructures, such as La Chureca landfill or the Sävenäs waste incinerator, constitute examples of what Foucault called more specifically heterotopic places of deviation: 'those in which individuals (and objects) whose behaviour is deviant in relation to the required mean or norm are placed' (Foucault, 1986: 25). Waste implies deviance per se: the disposed object no longer displays a function or utility for the person who cast it out. The deviant objects are placed in these heterotopic places in order to be transformed: reused, recycled in any material or as energy or simply stored. Society creates places such as prisons, cemeteries, landfill sites or incinerators, to contain and control threats to the well-functioning city. In these places, waste is stored, transformed, locked and often hidden until it flows towards new transformations along the waste management chain.

This leads to yet another function of waste urban infrastructures as heterotopic places that support the utopia of a well-functioning city. Waste urban infrastructures make possible functional urban life through the constant removal of waste that enables the city to be reborn and renewed everyday, ready to be used, produced and consumed everyday, as in Italo Calvino's (1974) invisible city of Leonia.

While the clean and sanitised city represents the utopic perfectly functioning city, waste urban infrastructures constitute the heterotopia of the city – the other city – making possible the utopia of the city of events, spectacles, business, leisure and consumption, to exist. Walter Benjamin identified the urban underworld with the urban Hell that exists underneath the heavenly urban environment (Buck-Morss, 1995). Every 'heaven requires its Hell in order to exist' (Kaika and Swyngedouw, 2000: 136). Likewise, the city of events and consumption requires unaesthetic, nasty, abject and stinky waste urban infrastructures to exist.

Economic growth in the city of Gothenburg demands the exactness and efficiency of the waste management system provided by the municipal waste corporation, and its high-technology facilities such as the Sävenäs incinerator – not only the collection and handling of waste, but also the production of energy such as as waste incineration. Similarly, the well-established events industry in Gothenburg requires the services of maintenance and repair of the city, such as the removal of tonnes of waste the day after each event. Even a 'hell on earth' such as La Chureca makes a fundamental contribution to the maintenance of the 'heavenly' parts of the city of Managua: the formal city and the city of the wealthy Managua society (Zapata Campos and Zapata, 2012). The illegal scavengers at La Chureca make an important contribution to the sustainability of the city by reducing the amount of waste finally disposed of in landfill, reducing greenhouse gas emissions and by recovering recyclables. La Chureca also enacts the invisible work carried out by scavengers for the international waste recycling industry, which represents a total value of over US$40 million (Carena, 2012). The export of recyclables from Nicaragua not only reaches countries in Latin America such as El Salvador and Guatemala, but also China and Europe, via Spain. In other words, the illegal work of scavengers carried out in indecent conditions supports the utopia of the city of Managua, and also wealthier societies elsewhere.

But how do waste infrastructures serve the urban condition? In the narratives collected in Gothenburg and Managua, waste urban infrastructures contributed to the utopia of the well-functioning city both by isolating and by hiding waste.

Isolating waste

Heterotopias, such as the waste urban infrastructures in Managua and Gothenburg, always have 'a system of opening and closing that isolates them and makes them penetrable' (Foucault, 1989: 26). Appropriately, La Chureca is located at the edge of Managua. La Chureca itself is a physically well-delimited and isolated site. To the north and east lies Lake Xolotlán and the contaminated Acahualinca Lagoon. To the west, the settlement is separated from the city by a long wall and a secondary road where some local non-governmental organisations (NGOs), providing some basic relief to the hard work of the scavengers, have built their headquarters. The main entrance, where the municipal waste trucks are weighed, provides a narrow access in the form of a tongue that goes deep into the rubbish dump to the south. The whole dump itself has turned into a rubbish mountain with a height of 20-30 metres, contributing to the intensity of its physical isolation (see Figure 3.4). Although less striking, in Gothenburg, the Tagene sanitary landfill site is also isolated. An electric fence protects copper and other sellable materials from theft, and the Sävenäs incinerator plant looks like a fortress, where the valuable waste fuel is protected and revalued after its transformation into clean energy (see Figure 3.5).

Figure 3.4: A mountain made of rubbish, La Chureca rubbish dump

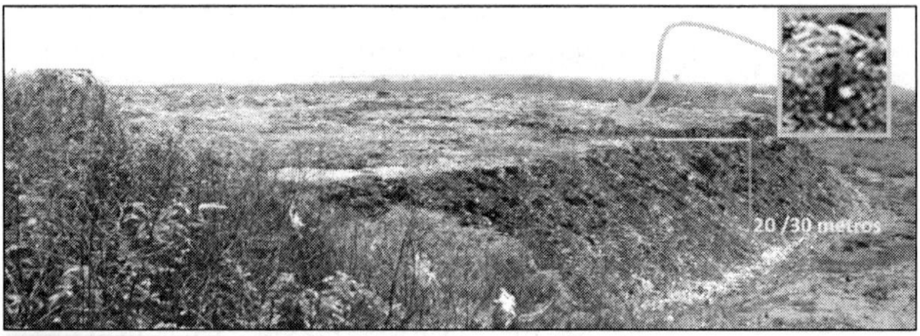

Source: Managa waste management office

Figure 3.5: Sävenäs waste incinerator, Gothenburg

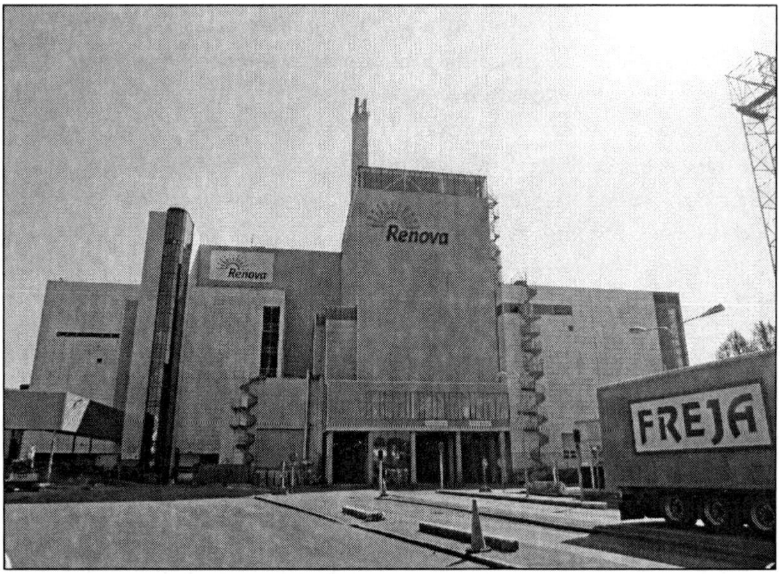

Only authorised staff are able to enter the impenetrable systems of heterotopic waste infrastructures. The waste room at Nordostpassagen is only accessible by municipal officers. Only municipal trucks and other authorised operators can, once waste is weighed and economic transactions done, enter La Chureca or the Sävenäs incinerator plant. The economic value as well as the potential risk of waste explains why a code, a key or a card become material intermediaries that protect and provide access to these places. Access to heterotopias, according to Foucault, may also be regulated by rites and purifications, such as the act of disposing of waste, which activates a chain of irreversible transition passages.

Predominant narratives, social constructions, beliefs and values are behind the regulation of the openings and closings of heterotopic places. In the narratives collected in Gothenburg and Managua, access was guaranteed by ideas such as the commodification of waste – its transformation into an attractive and valuable resource. At most of these infrastructures the weighing scale represented the entrance, where the economic transactions according to market prices of materials and energy were made, closely monitored by control offices, cameras or towers. Waste has to be paid for, to continue its flow and successive transformations. In other words, waste management in this waste governance regime (see Chapter Eight) also implies economic flows.

Hiding waste

In Gothenburg most of the waste infrastructures studied worked to hide waste: the container, the waste vacuum system, the waste truck, the waste incinerator at Sävenäs. In many European Nordic cities, the waste urban infrastructure has, by definition, been for decades the incinerator. In Gothenburg, the municipal waste managers presented the Sävenäs incinerator as the most efficient infrastructure to make waste disappear, reduced into slag, nanoparticles and a few CO^2 emissions. Reducing volume and transforming its material state represents the culmination of the process of dematerialisation and invisibilisation of waste. As noted above, waste managers described Sävenäs as a 'dioxin sink' of society.

In Managua, La Chureca was located at the edge of the city, far away from the eyes of the city dwellers, and in particular, the wealthy citizens. Even in the informal settlements, waste was cast out into roads, and riverbeds stored and hid waste, at least from the sight of those who dumped it. However, both in Gothenburg and Managua, the 'stubborn reminders of the materiality' (Kaika and Swyngedouw, 2000: 136) of waste were found. In La Chureca, waste was translated into disease caused by the ingestion of insalubrious food, the breathing of contaminated air or exposure to noxious substances. Disease attached itself and flourished as dengue, malaria and other plagues caused by poor housing conditions spread at La Chureca slum settlement and at the informal settlements in the *barrios* in Managua. In the *barrios* illegally dumped waste reappeared in spontaneous waste dumps. Even in the highly modern city of Gothenburg, wasted people (scavengers, homeless) and wasted things (urban litter) became visible eventually. Scavengers (see Figure 3.6) and waste container divers (see Figure 3.7) were observed salvaging recyclables and food from containers (Faktum, 2011).

Figure 3.6: Scavenger collects recyclables in the city of Gothenburg

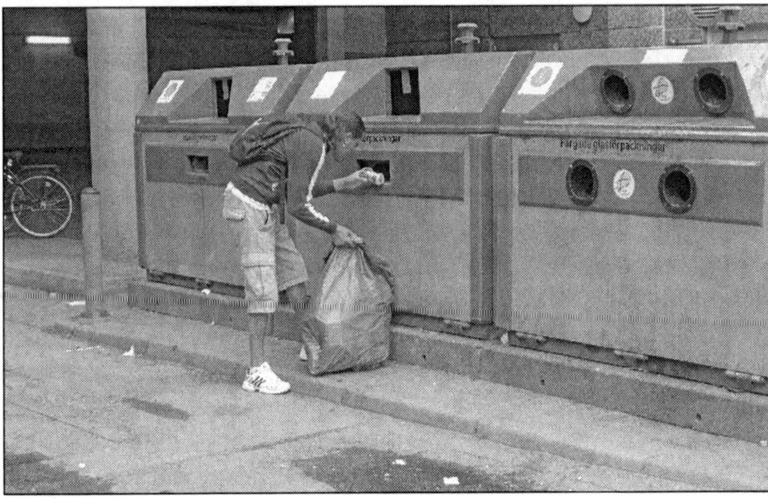

Implications for urban sustainable development

The question of where waste is locked and hidden, and from whom, brings up issues of power. Waste is hidden in waste infrastructures from wealthy and ordinary citizens, but is materially visible to, for example, scavengers, slum dwellers and other less well-off urban communities. Issues of environmental justice emerge in disclosing how deprived communities suffer the material effects of waste, waste infrastructures and even waste collection services (see Chapter Eleven). Or how the dispossessed and paupers surface from the city underworld or the city edge to extract the value left (as recyclable materials, but also as food or reusable objects) in what has already been cast out (see Chapter Nine). The sharp contrast of the heterotopia of waste in the city and the utopia of the clean, sanitised and well-functioning city reveals the contradictions of a sustainable urban development, of social and environmental justice in the city. The waste narratives presented in this chapter confirm that if you 'Study a city and neglect its sewers', or in this case, its waste urban infrastructures, 'you miss essential aspects of distributional justice and planning power' (Star, 1999: 379).

The opacity and inaccessibility of waste urban infrastructures, as of those studied in this chapter, contribute to obscure the social relations and power mechanisms through which the urbanisation of nature takes place in the city (Kaika, 2005) and along with the de-naturalisation of waste. Waste urban infrastructures are material mediators between nature and the city, where the flow of deterritorialised goods, materials and energy entering the city enact multiple transformations, finally

Figure 3.7: Waste container divers in Sweden

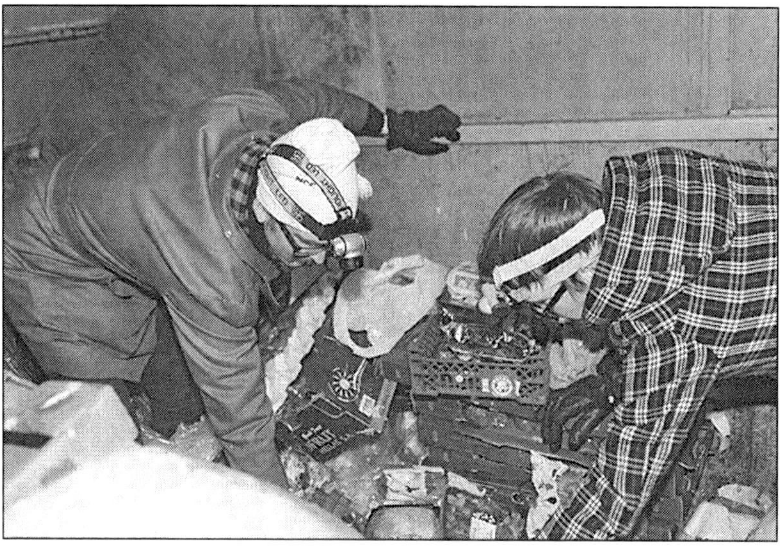

Copyright: Mario Prhat

becoming waste (Deleuze and Guattari, 1997). Or, in other words, making waste infrastructures invisible and inaccessible obscures the link between production, consumption and the disposal of waste. As a consequence, many city dwellers (for whom waste is hidden and inaccessible) find it difficult to couple their consumption habits with the growing mountain of waste – waste just disappears efficiently from their bins, shelves, fridges, drawers and wardrobes are empty again, ready to welcome new objects of consumption and renewal, just as in Italo Calvino's city of Leonia.

Therefore, one of the dilemmas facing the governance of cities towards more sustainable urban transformations is to what extent the heterotopic infrastructures that make waste efficiently disappear can paradoxically contribute to hide the steady growth of the overflow of waste. Or, differently expressed, how efficient heterotopias contribute to hide the consequences of the consumption and discard society.

Inverting waste infrastructures and opening up the heterotopias of the city

But how can we invert waste infrastructures and open up these heterotopic places to ordinary city dwellers? In the informal settlements in Managua, the transparency of technological, administrative and economic intermediaries has contributed to a visualisation of the exchange of waste, its connection with production, consumption and its transformation and implications. In the spontaneous settlements in Managua, householders themselves directly transfer waste to the waste collectors, unlike in most cities in the global North, where waste has become invisible, hidden from the moment it is disposed of in the waste room, from where it is collected, compressed into a sealed container into which not even the driver of the high-tech rubbish truck can see. In Managua, even the wastebag is emptied and reused. Waste is visible to the dwellers of the informal settlements but continues being invisible and odourless for the rich city dwellers who employ domestic staff to deal with their waste.

In 2010 Sweden saw waste quantities decrease for the second consecutive year (Swedish Waste Management, 2011); there was also a slow down of municipal waste production in European countries (Eurostat, 2011). While it is still too early to draw substantial conclusions, it is perhaps an indication of a hopeful decoupling between the production of material wealth and consumption and the production of waste in cities. During observations both in Gothenburg and Managua, a number of social practices and environmental policies were found that focused on inverting waste infrastructures: making waste visible and accessible. Recycling containers where waste was separated in Nordostpassagen succeeded in making visible the different materials and value still contained in waste. Waste trucks painted with the figurative waste they transported travelled daily through the city of Gothenburg, symbolically opening up their hidden and inaccessible contents for ordinary citizens to see. Waste collection invoices were sent to some neighbourhoods in Gothenburg, showing the exact weight of each waste amount produced by the householders and their corresponding price. Scholars visited both the Sävenäs incinerator and La Chureca dump, and were allowed to see and smell the material impacts of their consumption practices. Environmental campaigns, such as simulating the Ullevi football stadium in Gothenburg filling up with rubbish, attempted to show the volume of waste produced in the city (see Figure 3.8).

All these are attempts to unlock heterotopic infrastructures by visualising materially or symbolically the impacts of consumption practices. The governance of waste towards more sustainable urban transformations faces the challenge of opening up waste urban infrastructures, re-establishing the cognitive links between production, consumption and waste, breaking new roads towards 'wasting less' regimes (Corvellec and Hultman, 2012) and transforming these heterotopic places into transparent and unlocked containers of our outcasts.

Figure 3.8: Ullevi football stadium in Gothenburg, filled with rubbish

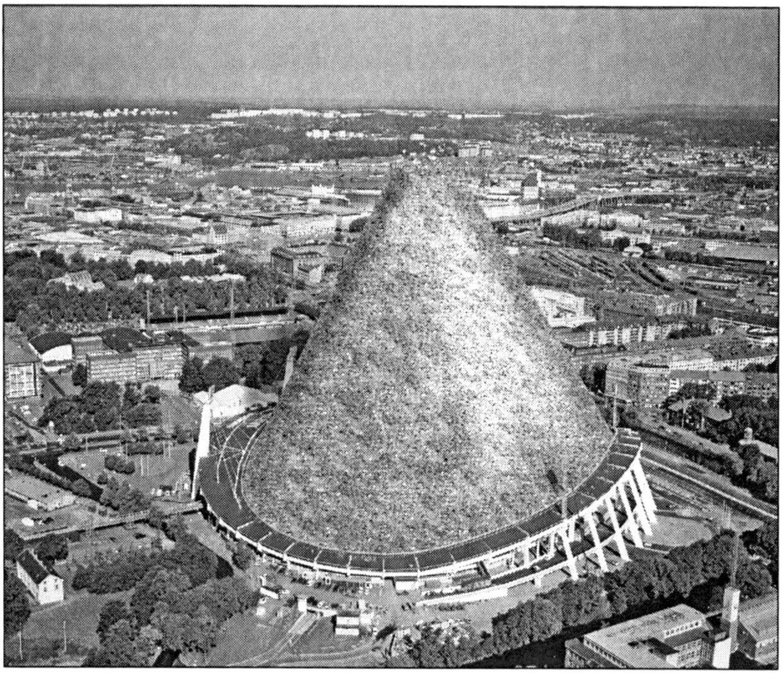

Source: Gothenburg waste management municipal office

Acknowledgements

This chapter is part of the research project 'Organising critical infrastructure services – A case study of waste management', funded by the Swedish Governmental Agency for Innovation Systems (VINNOVA), and research projects in Managua: 'Organising sustainability in the glocalised city', funded by the Jan Wallander Foundation and 'Waste in translation. How ideas of management travel from global to local', funded by the Gothenburg Centre for Globalisation and Development, University of Gothenburg.

References

Amin, A. and Graham, S. (1997) 'The ordinary city', *Transactions of the Institute of British Geographers*, vol 22, pp 411-29.

Bowker, G. and Star, S. (1989) *Sorting things out: Classification and its consequences*, Cambridge, MA: The MIT Press.

Buck-Morss, S. (1995) *The dialects of seeing: Walter Benjamin and the Arcades Project*, Cambridge, MA: The MIT Press.

Calvino, I. (1974) *Invisible cities* (translated by William Weaver), London: Secker & Warburg.

Carena (2011) *Waste management in Nicaragua*, Internal report, Managua: Carena.

Corvellec, H. and Hultman, J. (2012) 'From "less landfilling" to "wasting less" – Societal narratives, socio-materiality and organizations', *Journal of Organizational Change Management*, vol 44, no 10, pp 2413-27.

Deleuze, G. and Guattari, F. (1988) *A thousand plateaus: Capitalism and schizophrenia*, London: The Athlone Press.

Envac (2012) 'Envac brings sustainable waste collection to the world' (www.envacgroup.com).

Eurostat (2011) 'Generation and treatment of municipal waste', *Environment and Energy*, Brussels: Eurostat.

Faktum (2011) 'Containerdykare', 1 March, Gothenburg.

Foucault, M. (1986) 'Of other spaces', *Diacritics*, vol 16, pp 22-7.

Gothenburg Press (2011) *Skattehöjning öppnar ölslussen i Tyskland*, 5 September, Gothenburg: Göteborgs Posten (Gothenburg Press).

Graham, S. and Marvin, S. (2001) *Splintering urbanism: Networked infrastructures, technological mobilities and the urban condition*, London: Routledge.

Graham, S. and Thrift, N. (2007) 'Out of order: understanding repair and maintenance', *Theory, Culture & Society*, vol 24, no 1, pp 1-23.

Grigsby, V. (2008) 'The "new" Chureca: from garbage to human dignity', *Revista Envío*, vol 321, April (www.envio.org.ni).

Kaika, M. (2005) *City of flows: Modernity, nature, and the city*, New York: Routledge.

Kaika, M. and Swyngedouw, E. (2000) 'Fetishizing the modern city: The phantasmagoria of urban technological networks', *International Journal of Urban and Regional Research*, vol 24, no 1, pp 120-38.

Parés Barberena, M.I. (2006) *Estrategia municipal para la intervención integral de asentamientos humanos espontáneos de Managua Nicaragua*, CEPAL (Comisión Económica para América Latina y el Caribe), (ECLAC: Economic Commission for Latin America and the Caribbean) Managua: Naciones Unidas (*Municipal Strategy for integral planning of informal settlements in Managua, Nicaragua*) Naciones Unidas, United Nations.

Rathje, W. and Murphy, C. (2001) *Rubbish! The archaeology of garbage*, Tucson, AZ: The University of Arizona Press.

Renova (2011a) *Annual report*, Gothenburg: Renova.

Renova (2011b) *Annual environmental report*, Gothenburg: Renova.

Renova (2012) *From waste to clean energy*, Gothenburg: Renova (www.renova.se/Global/pdf/From_waste_to_clean_energy_light_web.pdf).

Robinson, J. (2006) *Ordinary cities: Between modernity and development*, London: Routledge.

Robinson, J. (2011) 'Cities in a world of cities: the comparative gesture', *International Journal of Urban and Regional Research*, vol 35, no 1, pp 1-23.

Star, S. (1999) 'The ethnography of infrastructure', *American Behavioral Scientist*, vol 43, pp 377-91.

Swedish Environmental Agency (2011) *From waste management to resource management: Sweden's waste plan 2012-2017*, Draft version 2011-09-12, Stockholm: Naturvårdsverket.

Swedish Waste Management (2011) 'Swedish waste management' (www.avfallsverige.se).

UNDP (United Nations Development Program) (2009) *Alianzas para el manejo de desechos sólidos en el Municipio de Managua*, (*Alliances for household solid waste management in the municipality of Managua*) Project document, Managua: UNDP.

Zapata Campos, M.J. and Zapata, P. (2012) 'Changing La Chureca. Organising city resilience through action nets', *Journal of Change Management*, vol 12, no 3, pp 323-37.

Zapata Campos, M.J. and Zapata, P. (2013) 'Switching Managua on! Connecting forgotten wastecapes to the city', *Environment and Urbanization*, vol 25, no 1, pp 225-42.

Part II

Global waste discourses and narratives shaping local practices

FOUR

When clean and green meets the Emerald Isle: contrasting waste governance narratives in Ireland and New Zealand

Anna Davies

Introduction

Although attention to waste governance has burgeoned over the last decade, progressing both theoretical understanding (see Bulkeley et al, 2007) and policy tool development (Hill et al, 2002), most of this work has focused either in-depth on one country or by examining particular mechanisms at a general level across widely varying nations or regions (see Parto, 2005). Both approaches have generated significant advances in understanding how governance practices *in toto* evolve in particular spaces, and how specific governing tools are applied through time and space, but neither provides extended comparative commentary. The aim of this chapter is, drawing on earlier comparative research (Davies, 2008a), to work with the insights gained from these existing waste governance approaches to undertake a detailed analysis of waste governance narratives and their influence over policy tools and waste management outcomes. Ireland and New Zealand have been selected for this purpose on the grounds that they share a degree of commonality in terms of population size, history and development. Both also accept the waste management hierarchy, which identifies waste prevention as the preferred option, then reuse, recycling and recovery, including energy recovery, with safe disposal as a last resort, as a guiding framework for sustainable waste management. More generally both are island nations that have faced significant challenges and conflicts over recent years in terms of how best to manage their waste. Of course there are also significant differences between the two nations that co-exist alongside these commonalities and, as the chapter outlines, even apparent similarities can conceal diverse experiences.

Initially the evolving pathways for political, cultural, economic and environmental development in the two countries are summarised and compared. The next section details the formal waste policy landscape of both countries, which is followed by an examination of the key governing interactions between the tiers and spheres of waste governance that appear to have influenced the policy landscape and the outcomes of those negotiated governing arrangements. The final section concludes with a reflection on the extent to which commonly articulated narratives, such as the waste management hierarchy, act as tools of convergence or obfuscation in relation to actual waste governance practices.

Governance landscapes

Despite being located in different hemispheres, there are some similarities between political and economic developments in both Ireland and New Zealand, not least that British colonialism has had a significant impact on both. Although the countries are now independent and have developed a parliamentary democracy, New Zealand remains part of the British Commonwealth while Ireland operates as an individual member state of a supra-national governing body, the European Union (EU). Internal government structures have also diverged in terms of the roles and responsibilities located at different scales. New Zealand is characterised by a devolved system that allocates regional and sub-regional (territorial) government significant powers. Ireland conversely has a local government structure that is lacking in influence and regional structures that play little part in most governing activities, although interestingly, new regional structures were developed for waste management in the 1990s, which will be addressed later in this chapter. The populations of both countries are broadly similar, with Ireland estimated to have a population of over 4.5 million in 2011 (CSO, 2011) and New Zealand just over 4 million in 2006 (Statistics New Zealand). More recent statistics are not available in New Zealand due to the earthquake in Christchurch in 2011 that meant that the national census was not held. The landmass of New Zealand is larger, however, leading to a relatively lower population density.

It has been argued that the legacy of colonialism has also shaped attitudes and approaches to natural resource management in both Ireland and New Zealand. In New Zealand issues related to environmental stewardship have been on the political agenda since the Treaty of Waitangi was signed in 1840. Concerns over the exploitation of natural resources by colonial settlers from this time led to a strong environmental movement, the formation of the world's first national Green Party in 1972, and arguably laid the foundations for the Resource Management Act (RMA) 1991. Heralded as a progressive environmental strategy at the time, the impacts of these developments have subsequently been contested, yet there remains a popular connection with the moniker of 'clean and green' for many New Zealanders to the present day.

While exploitation of the natural resource base in Ireland has also played a powerful role in the Irish psyche, the form and function has been very different. For many, identity with nature, and in particular 'the land', in Ireland can be traced back to the devastating potato famine in the mid-1800s and the political processes that compounded that phenomenon. Land values in Ireland were, as a result, often couched in utilitarian terms, with nature conservation and environmental regulation seen as a preoccupation of privileged, often urban, elites and an interference with private property rights. While public opinion surveys now suggest rising awareness of environmental issues, the development of an influential environmental movement at national and international levels has not emerged. Stimulus for improved environmental policy performance has, as a result, come predominantly from the EU. That said, the Irish Green Party (Comhaontas Glas), formed in 1981, has had members elected as TDs (Teachta Dála, or public representatives and members of the Dáil), and became a minority partner in the ruling coalition between 2007 and 2011. Green Party TDs held influential positions within the coalition with key posts for the environment: Minister for Environment, Heritage and Local Government; Minister for Communications, Energy and Natural Resources; and Minister of State for Food and Horticulture. Whether this led to any heightening of environmental concerns within government, particularly once the financial crisis broke in 2008, has yet to be rigorously demonstrated in any substantive sense. Certainly the new political administration has sought to distance itself and its policies from many of the environmental interventions set out by their predecessors.

In terms of direct environmental regulation, both countries have adopted the globally developed discourse of sustainable development as a guiding narrative for their strategies for more than a decade (MfE, 1995, 2003; DoELG, 1997, 2002), and a consolidation of regulatory frameworks has occurred during the same period. However, the ways in which sustainable development has been interpreted in both countries reflects the wider socioeconomic and political regimes in which the environmental regulations are situated.

With respect to environmental policy evolution then, there are similarities between the two countries in terms of a general commitment to sustainable development that has been largely characterised as ecologically modern in its formulation (Jackson and Dickson, 2007; Davies, 2009a, 2009b). However, Ireland has constructed a system of decision making and enforcement that is far more centralised than New Zealand, and this governance structure is repeated, to a large extent, in the field of waste management.

Governing waste

Policy interventions

With respect to waste management, the similarity of experience between Ireland and New Zealand, at least until the 1990s, is striking. A large proportion of municipal waste was disposed of to loosely regulated landfill sites that were run by local authorities for local communities. Neither country had extensive systems for recycling or large-scale facilities for municipal solid waste incineration. The regulatory framework, as with wider environmental controls, was a fragmented system of public health and local government acts that were widely recognised as insufficient to deal with increasing volumes and the complexity of waste.

New Zealand began restructuring its waste policy landscape by setting explicit targets for recycling in 1990, although these were subsequently dropped when progress towards attainment was slow. A waste management policy document published in 1992 instead emphasised the importance of attention to the waste management hierarchy in waste programmes. The waste management hierarchy also made an appearance in Ireland at a similar time stimulated by developments within the EU. By 1996 both countries had begun to formalise more sophisticated waste management planning regimes. In New Zealand this was achieved through an amendment to the Local Government Act while a specific Waste Management Act was developed in Ireland. Both systems called for the production of sub-national waste management plans for municipal solid waste. There was, however, more prescription regarding the waste planning process in Ireland, and the legislation provided for more central control over the nature and form of plans. In Ireland local authorities were required to come together in a regional structure to develop their plans (Davies, 2003). Similar calls for the regionalisation of waste plans are emerging in New Zealand, and a few such plans have recently been developed, but up until the Waste Minimisation Act 2008 detailed below, regional or local waste plans in New Zealand lacked the depth and detail of their Irish counterparts.

In New Zealand pressure to reconceptualise waste as a resource and to refocus attention higher up the waste management hierarchy gained momentum in 2006 with the production of a private members bill on waste minimisation. This was proposed by Nandor Tanczos, a Green Party Member of Parliament (MP). The publication of a government Cabinet Paper, *Towards a sustainable New Zealand: Measures to minimize solid waste* (MfE, 2007), marked a sea change of policy positioning with governmental support for a national waste levy and more regulation of voluntary initiatives.

The waste disposal levy not only functions as a financial instrument seeking to encourage alternative waste management behaviours; it also requires formal and regular data collection on waste disposal figures. Such waste information collection aims to improve monitoring and evaluation of policy interventions, and all registered facility operators have been collated since July 2009. There are opportunities to waive these fees as was done, for the first time, in November 2010 following the Canterbury earthquake. The levy revenue is split equally between local councils, on a population basis, who are required to spend the money on promoting or achieving waste minimisation in accordance with their Waste Management and Minimisation Plans (WMMPs) and the Waste Minimisation Fund that provides funding for waste minimisation projects. The impact of the act on waste management was so significant that the Ministry for the Environment published guidelines to promote good practice, and a new strategy reiterating the requirements was published in 2010 (MfE, 2010). This strategy states that '[w]hile the "zero waste" vision of the 2002 Strategy was ambitious, many of its targets were unable to be measured or achieved. The revised Strategy enables a more flexible approach to waste management and minimisation through two high level goals: reducing harm and improving efficiency' (MfE, 2010: 3). A preliminary review of the waste levy impact conducted in 2011 indicated no evidence of an increase in incidence or quantity of illegally dumped waste, although it was recognised that potential levy avoidance through misclassification of material diverted could take place. Insufficient evidence exists to accurately determine the extent of this levy avoidance at present.

European directives have fundamentally shaped waste policy in Ireland. In particular, the demands of the 1999 EU Waste Framework Directive and its subsequent revisions have required target setting for significant diversion of waste from landfill. A key milestone was the

Waste Management Act 1996 (and its subsequent amendment in 2001) which required extensive planning, inter-county cooperation and the development of levies for plastic bags and landfilled waste. In 2004 a review of waste management highlighted the need for user-based waste charges for household waste collections as a mechanism to send more accurate signals to consumers about the cost of waste management, and these became a requirement by 2005. Despite these developments, there were still concerns within government about meeting waste diversion targets set out by Europe, and the slow progress of incineration facilities was seen as a major obstacle here. In response, developments, including incinerators, considered to be of national importance were permitted to circumvent local planning processes through the Planning and Development (Strategic Infrastructure) Act in 2006. Whether this has actually speeded up decision making is unclear for while the first municipal solid waste incinerator came on stream in 2011 there has been no progress on other proposed facilities.

In 2009 a report on international waste practice was published as the basis for a review of national waste management policy in Ireland. From this a *Draft Statement of Waste Policy* was produced with the aim of ensuring that waste management services are 'delivered by the public and private sectors in an environmentally progressive and cost efficient manner' (Department of Environment, Community and Local Government, 2011). Although such a statement reiterates the ethos of the 1996 strategy, and its amendments, the major difference is greater encouragement to move waste management practices further up the waste management hierarchy, particularly with regard to biodegradable waste where current trajectories are not on track to meet EU targets. Since July 2010 producers of food waste at specified premises are required to segregate food waste and to ensure its collection and recovery by authorised collectors and facilities (DoEHLG, 2009: 11). The election of a new coalition government in 2011 caused a pause in the momentum behind the review of waste policy, but in April 2011 the new minister signalled his intention to fulfil many of the proposals in the draft review by 2012

Overall policy interventions in both countries have striking similarities and appear to be on a pathway of convergence around the need to progress further up the waste management hierarchy, and both seem to see the use of financial instruments as an integral part of achieving this. This commonality aside, there are significant organisational differences for delivering these goals. The centralised nature of policy making in Ireland is becoming more pronounced, while there are few signs that the strong local input into waste planning are being eroded in New Zealand. Equally there remains a commitment to investing in incineration in Ireland, arguably facilitated by the EU's ongoing requirement to divert land from landfill. Incineration, by contrast, has never been a feature of municipal waste management in New Zealand. Of course such policy evolution in both Ireland and New Zealand has not been generated without significant input from various stakeholders. The nature of interactions between stakeholders and decision makers and the extent of stakeholder influence on outcomes is, however, not always clearly visible by examining policy statements alone. The following section draws on material generated by interviews with a range of stakeholders integral to waste management in both countries in order to establish perceptions of interaction and influence in respective waste policy landscapes.

Stakeholder interactions

Patterns of interaction between, and the influence of, actors across tiers (from the transnational to local) and spheres (including private, public and civil society) of waste policy in both countries are dynamic. There are manifold opportunities for formal and informal negotiation of policy frameworks on an ongoing basis, and it is not possible to document these in any extended way here. Instead the aim is to compare the general ways in which different spheres and tiers of activity intersect in order to establish areas of commonality and divergence.

In Ireland and New Zealand the private sector is a dominant actor in waste management service delivery (Forfás, 2008). Municipal waste in Ireland is owned and operated by the public sector in only 28 per cent of cases, with the remainder either sub-contracted to the private sector (5 per cent) or a purely private affair (67 per cent). The figures are even more extreme in New Zealand, with only 10 per cent of collections entirely owned and operated by the public sector, a clear corollary of neoliberal reforms during the 1980s. Importantly, however, most of the private sector services in New Zealand are directly shaped by contracts with local authorities (80 per cent), a feature which is being proposed for Ireland in recent waste policy reviews. Interesting though they are in terms of comparing divergent delivery mechanisms, the figures do not reveal the nature of private sector contributions. In both cases there has been a consolidation of the waste industry with the emergence of large waste companies, sometimes international companies, controlling significant elements of the waste stream. In Ireland the private sector, albeit a different arm of it, has also played a major role in the formation of waste management plans. The Waste

Management Act 1996 required local authorities to seek assistance from waste experts when drafting their waste plans due to concerns over levels of expertise at the local level across Ireland. The waste experts employed in this role were entirely drawn from the private consultancy sector. Equally, environmental consultancies (the same companies in some cases) have been pivotal in developing and providing waste awareness initiatives both at a national scale (Race Against Waste) and sub-nationally (for example. the Dublin waste-to-energy project). Waste plans and waste awareness campaigns in New Zealand, by contrast, have been very much driven by local authorities, often with assistance from civil society groups (Davies, 2008a)

Civil society actors have played more divergent roles in waste management in Ireland and New Zealand. Until recently Ireland's waste related civil society organisations – be that community based recycling organisations, anti-incineration campaigns or organised protests surrounding waste charges – have been few in number, weakly networked and generally marginalised from decision making circles (Davies, 2007; 2008b). However, community based reuse organisations, while still a small sector of around 10 enterprises, are seeking to establish a stronger national voice with the formation of the all-Ireland Community Reuse Network in 2010. The civil society sector in New Zealand has many more community resource or recycling organisations that provide a whole range of services and contribute significantly to the delivery of local waste management strategies in particular areas. These groups communicate and collaborate through a variety of networks, such as Zero Waste New Zealand and the Community Recycling Network that listed 30 community groups as members on their website in 2011, that provide a national voice for their concerns in policy debates. The influence of these organisations can be seen directly in the fact that zero waste was included in the New Zealand waste strategy in 2002, however, actors from all governing spheres have commented that this was more of a rhetorical statement than a real commitment to zero waste at the time (Davies, 2008a). There is not one technical definition of zero waste, although the Zero Waste Alliance in 2004 defined it as:

> ... a goal that is ethical, economical, efficient and visionary, to guide people in changing their lifestyles and practices to emulate sustainable natural cycles, where all discarded materials are designed to become resources for others to use. Zero Waste means designing and managing products and processes to systematically avoid and eliminate the volume

> and toxicity of waste and materials, conserve and recover all resources, and not burn or bury them. Implementing Zero Waste will eliminate all discharges to land, water or air that are a threat to planetary, human, animal or plant health.

So, despite the devolved system of government in New Zealand, there exists a strong national base within the waste civil society sector. Yet in Ireland, where the governing system is solidly centralised, there is limited (albeit growing) national organisation. One reason for the divergence may be located in the histories of environmental activism within two different countries. It has been suggested that popular environmental protest in Ireland has been dominated by localised community responses to discrete environmental threats (Leonard, 2007), whereas there has been much more of a campaigning tradition focused on broad natural resource management issues in New Zealand (see Pawson and Brooking, 2002). This attention to issues of resource stewardship may be linked to the influence of Māori culture (Kaitiatanga) as enshrined, but also contested, within policy making through the Treaty of Waitangi in combination with the particular nature–society relations that have emerged since the European settlement. Equally, the lack of a strong nationwide environmental movement in Ireland may also be linked to particular conceptions of nature–society relations that have been coloured by past periods of colonialism (Gilmartin, 2009).

While it is clear that waste management practices exhibit features associated with a system of governance in both countries, with neoliberal reforms in New Zealand devolving power downwards and outwards beyond central state departments and an increasingly privatised waste collection system in Ireland, it is the case that the public sector retains directive power. Ireland's central government supports a fervently ecologically modern agenda with environmental problems seen as primarily technical and economic rather than social or political (Davies and Mullin, 2011). While similar rhetorical devices are used in a New Zealand context, the central state is far less prescriptive, and it is local government that is charged with setting planning agendas and steering private sector activities through sub-contracting mechanisms. Having said this it seems there are moves, through the Waste Minimisation Bill 2008, to reclaim at least some tighter central government control over waste governance tools, particularly, for example, through accreditation of voluntary product stewardship schemes.

At the same time as being less prescriptive, the Ministry for Environment in New Zealand is perceived as being more open to discussions with civil society organisations concerned with environmental issues generally and waste matters specifically. Despite the existence of formal partnership agreements on social policy between the state, employers, farmers, unions and the community in Ireland since 1987, a specific environment pillar was not included in discussions until 2009. Of course access does not necessarily equate to influence in terms of policy negotiation or implementation, and nor do actors from different spheres of governance necessarily want to be considered as identical organisations. For example, it was a concern of civil society groups in New Zealand that their activities in terms of waste management were considered the same as the private sector, despite the added environmental and social benefits they provided. In addition, while the RMA incorporates opportunities for public participation, it has been argued that the effects-based focus and legalistic framework of the RMA actually serves to subtly oppress participation of those without institutional or corporate experience (Gunder and Mouat, 2002), and such criticisms might equally be levelled at participatory mechanisms in an Irish context.

The form of waste policy interventions in Ireland and New Zealand is clearly shaped by a complex of historical and contemporary relationships between actors and agencies from all spheres of governance at different scales. The form of these interactions is not fixed, but evolves continuously through formal and informal lobbying and negotiation. The next section of this chapter considers how the particular forms of interactive interventions have affected the landscape of waste itself in both countries.

Narratives, mechanisms and impacts

There are many deliberations in policy literature about how to evaluate the success or otherwise of particular policy interventions (Crabbé and Leroy, 2008). There is not scope in this section to reiterate these enduring debates in any general sense, save to rehearse the truism that the multiple interests involved in, and affected by, policy interventions provide many definitions of success. In this section these issues are side-stepped to some extent by a focus on the outcomes of the policy interventions. Outcomes are here defined as the discourses or narratives that are developed to conceptualise waste, the policy mechanisms institutionalised to manage waste and, more materially, the impact that those discourses and mechanisms have on the nature and volumes of waste being produced. In terms of waste narratives (see also Chapters Five and Eight, this volume), central governments in both Ireland and New Zealand are rhetorically wedded to the waste management hierarchy. The recent revisions to this hierarchy emphasising waste minimisation as defined by the EU Waste Framework Directive are clearly permeating waste policies in both countries. Interestingly New Zealand is more advanced in this regard with the formalisation of the Waste Management and Minimisation Bill 2008, while Ireland produced its revised waste policy 'A resource Opportunity' only in July 2012. The impact of enforceable targets for EU member states for the diversion of waste from landfill, and specifically biodegradable waste, has tended to focus debates in Ireland around incremental moves up the hierarchy away from landfill. In contrast to New Zealand, this has brought the issue of waste incineration (as energy recovery and hence one step up the waste management hierarchy from disposal) to the fore in Ireland. So while there might appear to be discursive harmony in overarching waste narratives at a general level, there are quite different interpretations of the means and motivations just beneath the surface.

While the waste management hierarchy is the dominant narrative in both countries, there have been some important sub-narratives. Zero waste is a key example here. The language of zero waste has been used by civil society organisations and promoted by Zero Waste New Zealand since 1999. In 2001 40 per cent of local authorities in New Zealand had committed to achieve zero waste to landfill by 2015 or 2020 in their waste management plans. By 2006 this had increased to 70 per cent (51 out of 71 councils). A key victory for the zero waste movement was the inclusion of the term in the 2002 New Zealand waste strategy, 'towards zero waste and sustainable development'. However, by 2010 and the publication of the revised waste strategy, mention of zero waste was referred to historically as a 'vision' that was 'ambitious', with many of its targets 'unable to be measured or achieved' (MfE, 2010: 3). In Ireland zero waste has failed to make an impact on policy rhetoric, even though a zero waste organisation was formed in 1999 (Zero Waste Alliance Ireland). Indeed, a past Minister for the Environment is recorded as saying,

> ... those advocating a zero waste policy have zero credibility.... Had the Government adopted such an approach in our regional waste management plans, Ireland's waste management capability would be in a sorry state today, people would be paying more in taxes and foreign investors would not come to Ireland. (DoEHLG 2004: 5)

In contrast to zero waste, the private sectors in both countries, and also the public sector in Ireland, are far more comfortable with the sub-narrative of Integrated Solid Waste Management (ISWM). ISWM is characterised as a strategy that draws on a range of systems and processes to manage waste. As a result, all methods of waste management, including resource recovery and landfill, are viable options provided attention is paid to environmental impacts. Key within the ISWM schema are notions of efficiency, competitiveness, practicality and balance. These ideas are encapsulated in the annual waste benchmarking report of Forfás, Ireland's policy advisory board for enterprise, trade, science, technology and innovation, which states 'a key challenge for waste policy in Ireland is to balance economic and environmental goals in a way which will minimise business costs and avoid putting jobs at risk' (Forfás, 2010: 3).

The relative influence of waste narratives can be distilled from the mechanisms that have been developed to implement waste policies. Ireland introduced detailed legislation, the Waste Management Act 1996 (and amendments), that explicitly refers to the waste management hierarchy and calls for waste management planning regions to adopt an integrated waste management approach. In practice, the major outcomes of this mechanism have been the development of a recycling infrastructure across the country and plans for the development of municipal solid waste incinerators in particular locations. A combination of targets, levies and charges were introduced at the turn of the millennium in an attempt to shape waste practices (Davies and O'Callaghan-Platt, 2008). Only limited voluntary mechanisms such as REPAK, which is concerned with packaging waste, and the Race Against Waste awareness campaign have been developed to assist in the achievement of national policy statements. Waste minimisation only appeared on the policy radar in 2004 with the launch of the national waste prevention programme, run by the Environmental Protection Agency, which initiated its first phase of projects funded in 2006. In 2011 the Agency claimed that the programme had been cited as best practice by the EU Commission and the Organisation for Economic Co-operation and Development (OECD), although there are no details of such statements provided, and the OECD review of Ireland's environmental performance concluded that there was a need to 'reinvigorate implementation of the National Waste Prevention Programme' (OECD, 2010: 86).

New Zealand has likewise seen multiple developments in mechanisms to deal with waste since the 2002 national waste management strategy was published. Unlike Ireland there was no consideration of incineration as a means to reduce waste to landfill, although technically under the RMA a developer could propose an incinerator. It remains the general perception that incineration is unlikely in the New Zealand waste stream because of: a strong opposition lobby that includes a coalition of farming, environmental and community groups; adequate landfill capacity for the immediate short to medium term; and no supra-national level of government imposing enforceable targets for diversion from landfill. Nonetheless, waste policy developments in New Zealand and Ireland appear to be on a path of convergence in recent years. With the Waste Minimisation Bill 2008 New Zealand is beginning to embrace more market-based financial instruments such as the landfill levy. At the same time Ireland, encouraged by OECD and Forfás reviews, is seeking to extend its voluntary producer responsibility initiatives, a mechanism that New Zealand has adopted for some time.

Comparing outcomes of waste policy would be incomplete without attention to the material characteristics of waste itself. Such comparisons, however, require comparable data that are accurate and up-to-date. A deficiency in basic waste statistics was identified in both countries during the 1990s, and New Zealand produced its first national waste data report in 1997, with Ireland doing likewise in 1998. Since this time the Environmental Protection Agency in Ireland has reported on waste generation and management at regular intervals and most recently in 2011 (EPA, 2011a), but New Zealand has not conducted another national waste data collection exercise. The requirement on local authorities to collate and report on waste statistics within their local area, as directed by the Waste Minimisation Bill as part of the landfill levy, should help resolve some of the knowledge deficit. However, even in 2010 the Ministry for the Environment in New Zealand found that '[t]he lack of data about waste hampers our ability to plan appropriate activities to improve waste management and minimisation' (MfE, 2010: 3).

Bearing in mind the data limitations, the estimates of the amount of waste going to landfill from the two countries suggest that New Zealand sends around 2.5 million tonnes of waste to landfill (MfE, 2011), while Ireland reports just over 1.7 million tonnes (EPA, 2011b). While this suggests that Ireland's emphasis on diversion from landfill has been successful in quantifiable terms, the figures need to be read in the light of the dramatic economic downturn. The Environmental Protection Agency report highlights that the tonnage of waste to landfill has declined by 11 per cent since 2008, while the OECD suggests that economic growth and waste production have not been decoupled in Ireland (OECD, 2010). Given the lack of decoupling, any revival in economic growth will make attainment of EU targets even more challenging. There also remain 19 per cent of households in Ireland who do not avail of a waste collection service and whose waste cannot therefore be accurately accounted for. Overall evaluations of Ireland's waste practice are mixed with some good progress towards EU targets for recycling, but some outstanding risk that EU Landfill Directive targets for diversion of biodegradable municipal waste will not be attained by the deadlines of 2013 and 2016. Certainly the new EU Waste Framework Directive will continue to enact significant influence on the shape of waste management practices in Ireland over the next decade

Recent waste policy interventions in New Zealand mark a more radical departure from previous practices than Ireland. Concerns of non-governmental organisations (NGOs) regarding weak central leadership, variable local expertise and regulation appear to have finally caught the ear of the Ministry for the Environment. The revised waste strategy states that '[a]lthough there have been considerable improvements in access to recycling services and environmental controls around disposal facilities, waste management and minimisation practices still vary around the country and further improvements can be made' (MfE, 2010: 3). The impact of the Waste Minimisation Act is likely to take a few years to filter through, but already the waste levy generated around NZ$6 million that was distributed in the 2010–11 funding round to more than 20 projects.

Conclusion

This chapter adopted a comparative governance framework to explore evolving narratives of municipal solid waste policy in Ireland and New Zealand in relation to policy interventions, stakeholder interactions and outcomes. While this has revealed a patchwork of commonality and difference across the two countries, a convergence of language and approaches seems to be in the ascendance (see Table 4.1). This convergence is predominantly based on a common perception, at least among public and private waste actors, that waste is as much a business as it is a service. Linked to this business-oriented agenda are the twin drivers of efficiency and competitiveness, alongside a commitment to economies of scale and belief in a technical fix to waste management challenges. In this context the rhetorically flexible concept of integrated solid waste management is appealing to both public and private sector actors in the waste field exactly because it is not prescriptive about the 'best' means to deal with waste, and admits a range of tools and outcomes justified on the grounds of locally specific conditions. That this permits business as usual in waste management practices on the grounds of contextual conditions is clearly both a main part of its appeal for many, but is also seen as a major weakness among those arguing for more progressive and transformative approaches to waste. The waste management hierarchy, in contrast, has a more normative agenda in that there is a clear statement about optimal waste management practices (prevention and minimisation over disposal and resource recovery, for example). However, within the EU, the linearity of the waste management hierarchy and the setting of targets to divert waste from the least desirable management options (for example, landfill) has led to only incremental transitions in waste production. The more progressive narrative of zero waste has had a more volatile existence in Ireland and New Zealand, with initially positive and visible exposure in New Zealand before a gradual fading from

Table 4.1: Comparative waste governance: New Zealand and Ireland

Governing dimension	Ireland	New Zealand
Governing landscape	Independent parliamentary democracy Influential supra-national government (EU) Strong central government Utilitarian land ethic	Independent parliamentary democracy Autonomous nation state (British Commonwealth) Devolved government, strong regional government Resource stewardship
Waste landscape		
Pre-1990s	Weak, fragmented local government acts Predominance of landfill	Weak, fragmented local government acts Predominance of landfill
Post-1990s	Constructed regionalism (newly established waste regions based on agglomerated county government) Strong central government waste planning requirements (driven by EU directives) Improved recycling facilities Development of incineration (resource recovery) Enhanced utilisation of economic tools (plastic bag levy, landfill levy, pay-by-use waste charges) Formalised waste data collection	Strong regionalism (based on existing sub-national government structures) Weak central government guidance Zero waste Emergent voluntary agreements Limited economic tools Limited data collection
Emergent trends	Increasing privatisation (both policy and practice) Incremental change driven by strong external drivers Economic efficiency, practicality, competitiveness and balance	Waste minimisation Greater central government control Enhanced information collection Autonomy (with need for international credibility) Emergence of economic tools

public profile. In Ireland the movement has been pivotal in providing support and expertise in relation to anti-incineration movements, but the concept has not become broadly adopted, even within grassroots waste enterprises. Nonetheless waste governance arrangements in both countries are underpinned by a complex of historically grounded and culturally specific conditions in relation to resource management. For example, the widely articulated stewardship narrative of New Zealand creates connections with natural resources in ways that are not present in the psyche of mainstream Ireland, where a utilitarian land ethic dominates.

Perhaps it is unsurprising that, given the broader privatisation and translocalisation of waste practices driven increasingly by multinational waste management companies, the ideological ethos of zero waste has not found favour within mainstream waste management environments in either country. Yet a reflection on the ways that waste management practices have evolved since the 1990, suggests that wider discourses of environmental management and governance might be more influential in shaping waste management practices than the waste narratives that are invoked. For example, there is little evidence, in the revisions of waste policy that have recently emerged in New Zealand and in Ireland, that there is serious appetite among public and private waste actors for radical change to waste matters that might aim towards the pinnacle of the waste management hierarchy. Incremental improvements to recycling facilities, extended producer responsibility agendas and more nuanced fiscal instruments aimed at recovering the costs of waste management are prevalent, and are all deeply situated within the realm of traditional ecological modernisation where the main focus is a win-win for the economy and the environment. Equally, the financial conditions under which Ireland currently operates, as dictated by the guidelines set down by the troika of the International Monetary Fund (IMF), the European Central Bank and the European Commission, means that driving forces in operating any public service are efficiency and fiscal austerity. Such drivers are clearly shaping governmental actions at national and sub-national level, and the waste sector is no exception, reinforcing already existing trends towards more economic instruments and enhanced privatisation of the waste stream. As such, waste governing mechanisms are intimately related to broader trends in governance. In New Zealand this manifests itself in terms of devolved waste governance to regional and territorial authorities, which means that within broad parameters, waste management can be highly variable in different locations. The heavily prescribed nature of regional waste planning in Ireland, and the influential shaping forces of environmental consultants (with one consultant producing the majority of regional plans across the country), led to more consistent plans across the country, but the actual practice of waste management is increasingly shaped by the private sector companies that collect and dispose of waste.

This chapter has drawn together the experiences of waste management in Ireland and New Zealand that exhibit a number of common general characteristics, but which articulate different discourses around waste issues and adopt contrasting positions in relation to certain waste management practices. More detailed analysis suggests that explanations for these divergent pathways, both discursive and material, are rooted in a complex intertwining of political, economic, social and environmental histories in the two countries. Examining the respective roles that tiers of government and spheres of governance play in the waste management of both countries further accounts for the existence of contrasting waste practices, but it is the distinct geographies of multilevel government that stand out as the most significant area of contrast between the two cases, suggesting that while without doubt waste governance exists, government still matters.

Acknowledgements

This chapter draws on research conducted since 2001 that has been supported by a range of organisations, including the Environmental Protection Agency and the Irish Research Council for Humanities and Social Sciences.

References

Bulkeley, H., Watson, M., Hudson, R. and Weaver, P. (2007) 'Modes of governing municipal waste', *Environment and Planning A*, vol 39, no 11, pp 2733-53.

Crabbé, A. and Leroy, P. (2008) *The handbook of environmental policy evaluation*, London: Earthscan.

CSO (Central Statistics Office) (2011) *Census 2011 Results*, Dublin: CSO.

Davies, A.R. (2003) 'Waste wars – public attitudes and the politics of place in waste management strategies', *Irish Geography*, vol 36, no 1, pp 77-92.

Davies, A.R. (2007) 'A wasted opportunity? Civil society and waste management in Ireland', *Environmental Politics*, vol 16, no 1, pp 52-72.

Davies, A.R. (2008a) *Geographies of garbage governance: Interventions, interactions and outcomes*, Aldershot: Ashgate.

Davies, A.R. (2008b) 'Civil society activism and waste management in Ireland: the Carranstown anti-incineration campaign', *Land Use Policy*, vol 25, no 2, pp 161-72.

Davies, A.R. (2009a) 'Does sustainability count? Environmental policy, sustainable development and the governance of grassroots sustainability enterprise in Ireland', *Sustainable Development*, vol 17, no 3, pp 174-82.

Davies, A.R. (2009b) 'Clean and green? A governance analysis of waste management in New Zealand', *Journal of Environmental Planning and Management*, vol 52, no 2, pp 157-77.

Davies, A. and Mullin, S. (2011) 'Greening the economy: interrogating sustainability innovations beyond the mainstream', *Journal of Economic Geography*, vol 11, no 5, pp 793-816.

Davies, A.R. and O'Callaghan-Platt, A. (2008) 'Does money talk? Waste charging in the Republic of Ireland: government, governance and performance', *Journal of Environmental Policy and Planning*, vol 10, no 3, pp 1-17.

Department of Environment, Community and Local Government (2011) *Draft statement of waste policy: For consultation*, Dublin: Department of Environment, Community and Local Government.

DoELG (Department of the Environment and Local Government) (1997) *Sustainable development: A strategy for Ireland*, Dublin: DoELG.

DoELG (2002) *Making Ireland's development sustainable*, Dublin: DoELG.

DoEHLG (Department of the Environment, Heritage and Local Government) (2004) *Waste management – Taking stock and moving forward*, Dublin: DoEHLG.

DoEHLG (2009) *International review of waste management policy: Summary report*, Dublin: DoEHLG.

EPA (Environmental Protection Agency) (2011a) *National waste report 2009*, Wexford: EPA.

EPA (2011b) A *review of the Environmental Protection Agency*, Wexford: EPA.

Forfás (2008) Waste management benchmarking analysis and policy priorities, Dublin: Forfás.

Forfás (2010) *Waste management in Ireland: Benchmarking priorities and update 2010*, Dublin: Forfás.

Gilmartin, M. (2009) 'Border thinking: Rossport, Shell and the political geographies of a gas pipeline', *Political Geography*, vol 28, no 5, pp 274-82.

Gunder, M. and Mouat, C. (2002) 'Symbolic violence and victimization in planning processes: a reconnoitre of the New Zealand Resource Management Act', *Planning Theory*, vol 1, no 2, pp 124-45.

Hill, J., Bégin, A. and Shaw, B. (2002) *Creative policy packages for waste: Lessons for the UK*, London: Green Alliance.

Jackson, T. and Dixon, J. (2007) 'The New Zealand Resource Management Act: an exercise in delivering sustainable development through an ecological modernisation agenda', *Environment and Planning B: Planning and Design*, vol 34, no 1, pp 107-20.

Leonard, L. (2007) 'Environmentalism in Ireland: Ecological modernisation versus populist rural sentiment', *Environmental Values*, vol 16, no 4, pp 463-83.

MfE (Ministry for the Environment) (1995) *Environment 2010*, Wellington: MfE.

MfE (2003) *Sustainable development: Programme of action*, Wellington: MfE.

MfE (2007) *Towards a sustainable New Zealand: Measures to minimize solid waste*, Wellington: MfE.

MfE (2010) *New Zealand waste management strategy*, Wellington: MfE.

MfE (2011) *Work Programme – Waste*, Wellington: MfE.

OECD (Organisation for Economic Co-operation and Development) (2010) *OECD environmental performance reviews. Ireland: Conclusions and recommendations*, Paris: OECD.

Parto, S. (2005) *Good governance and policy analysis*, Maastricht: MERIT-Infonomics Research Memorandum Series.

Pawson, E. and Brooking, T. (eds) (2002) *Environmental histories of New Zealand*, Oxford: Oxford University Press.

FIVE

Waste in translation: global ideas of urban waste management in local practice

Patrik Zapata

Introduction

The multiplicity of global actors leads to a variety of ideas on what sustainable waste management is and should be. Global organisations bring with them their definitions, problematisations, policies, plans, technologies and management models on how to handle waste locally. The local practice is therefore affected considerably by global organisations, especially in the global South where global actors are often represented via development programmes in which global ideas are promoted and proposed.

Managua, Nicaragua, is a local representation of such a multiplicity of global actors. In Managua, six out of seven development projects carried out by the local government in 2010 and 2011 (co-funded by international aid development organisations) were related to waste management (Zapata Campos and Zapata, 2012a), and a diversity of ideas are told and acted out in Managua. One of the global actors that states its ideas on sustainable waste management is UN-Habitat (2010a). In Managua UN-Habitat are running a project dealing with the improvement of solid waste management in the city.

The glocalisation of development aid cannot be reduced to the simple compliance, assimilation and appropriation of programmes transferred from North to South. Instead, development aid projects are also locally contested and eventually localised (see, for example, Rossi, 2006; Sulle, 2010; Zapata Campos and Zapata, 2012b), often overtly or silently. However interesting, that is not the theme of this chapter. Instead, the subject of analysis in this chapter is the global ideas on waste management formulated by UN-Habitat and the local waste management practices they promote. The chapter aims to explore some of the many views on waste management as an issue of global and local governance of sustainability based on the question: what are the global ideas, and which views on sustainable waste management do they entail?

After a note on methodology, the chapter presents the ideas on waste and waste management that are promoted by UN-Habitat globally and locally. Second, the global and local levels are compared and the extent to which they do or do not accord with each other is discussed and, based on a close reading of the local texts, the chapter discusses what views and ideas on sustainable waste management are presented and practised in Managua, and their implications for the view on how waste is organised.

A close reading of waste management texts

By means of deconstruction, assumptions, categorisations, distinctions and conflicts hidden in a text can be brought to attention, questioned and discussed, for example, the assumption that men constitute the norm in organisations, or for that matter, that waste management is strictly physical. Analysis in this chapter is inspired by Martin (1990), and the strategies for deconstructing texts she introduced to organisation studies. More specifically, the focus of the analysis is on dichotomies, underlying assumptions, false distinctions, multiple meanings and contradictions found in two studies: (1) a document that presents and summarises the UN-Habitat waste management project in Managua; and (2) an excerpt from *Solid waste management in the world's cities* (UN-Habitat, 2010a), where UN-habitat presents its views on sustainable waste management at a global level. The results are then compared.

It should also be mentioned that the author has a pre-understanding of the projects the texts represent and their context. This chapter is part of a research project, 'Waste in translation', in which María José Zapata Campos and the author conducted two field visits to Managua during December 2009 to February 2010 and January to February 2011. During fieldwork personal interviews were conducted with 60 key actors related to La Chureca and six externally funded development projects regarding waste management in Managua. Field research also included non-participant observation over a multitude of meetings and events during the implementation of the projects, photography and the writing of a field diary. Some of the texts produced during interviews and observations are used to illustrate the analysis presented in this chapter.

Global ideas on waste management

UN-Habitat is the United Nations (UN) agency for human settlements, responsible for promoting more sustainable urbanisation, a field where it 'must play a leadership and catalytic role' (UN-Habitat, 2008). To do that, UN-Habitat hosts workshops and conferences, develops organisational tools and training material, and by collecting lessons learned and best practice, aims to 'help policy-makers and local communities get to grips with the human settlements and urban issues and find workable, lasting solutions' (UN-Habitat, 2012). With the publication of *Solid waste management in the world's cities* (2010a), UN-Habitat aims to 'capture the world's current waste management trends … and provide a reference point for managing solid waste in the world's cities and towns' (2010a: v). In the book, UN-Habitat presents experiences and data from 20 reference cities (one of them is Managua), and reflects on key elements in and how Integrated Solid Waste Management (ISWM) can be achieved. For this chapter, these key elements are what represent global ideas on sustainable waste management, and they are summarised below:

- *Different approaches to local problems:* every city is different, and furthermore, the solid waste management systems are in different development stages. Therefore, all efforts to improve the system have to be grounded locally. '[T]he best solution in one location may not be the most appropriate somewhere else' (UN-Habitat, 2010a: 205).
- *Data is power: indicators of good practice:* 'If a city aspires to a "modern" waste management system, then a good data collection and management system need to be seen as a key component' (UN-Habitat, 2010a: 207).
- *Consider all dimensions of integrated, sustainable waste management:* good practice in the 20 cities focuses on the physical elements of waste management, as collection, disposal and resource recovery. However, 'Inclusivity, involving both the users and the service provider is a key feature in all the examples, as is progress in developing sound institutions and proactive policies' (UN-Habitat, 2010a: 207).
- *Building recycling rates:* 'The informal sector is clearly any city's ally – if the city had to deal with these quantities [that the informal actors pick, upgrade and trade] as waste, then their costs would rise dramatically' (UN-Habitat, 2010a: 208). By handling the waste, the informal sector is 'providing a "sink" for the waste, that the city otherwise would have to pay for' (UN-Habitat, 2010a: 208). By working with the informal recyclers, providing them space and

legitimacy, the city brings them into the formal economy, potentially increasing their living standards and the recycling rates.

- *A focus on waste reduction:* there is a shift from a focus on recycling to waste prevention, not only in the most developed countries, due to population growth, migration and increasing standards, but also in the less developed (of the 20) cities. Therefore, an ISWM approach is likely to come at the problem from three directions at the same time:

    1. from the 'bottom', to get onto the hierarchy in the first place by phasing out open dumps;
    2. from the 'middle', ensuring that wasters are increasingly diverted from disposal to reuse, recycling, organics, valorisation and composting, and;
    3. from the 'top', to reduce waste source and to bring waste growth under control so that a city can make real progress (UN-Habitat, 2010a: 209).

The key conclusion, and hence the main advice, of the book is: 'a sustainable local solution must be acceptable, appropriate and affordable in the local circumstances' (UN-Habitat, 2010a: 212).

- *Use all available sources of finance:* the key conclusion points directly to a dilemma regarding external financing in developing countries. If the waste management system (or parts of it) is upgraded to meet international standards, it is most often not affordable for the city, or if they can afford the initial investment, the running costs are too high, or the city might have to take out loans and thus risk getting caught in a debt trap. As UN-Habitat writes:

> ... neither international financial institutions, nor national governance structures are geared to this "pick-and-mix" approach. IFIs [international financial institutions] and their governing boards need to look again at their policies, particularly at their insistence on "international standards" as a condition for financing ... it seems unreasonable to insist that the same standards form part of the next step in every developing country as a condition for providing financial assistance. (UN-Habitat, 2010a: 212)

Rather, UN-Habitat propose that one should prioritise 'capacity- and knowledge-building in order to develop inclusive approaches, sound institutions and proactive policies, and to work towards financial sustainability' (UN-Habitat, 2010a: 212).

Locally practised ideas of sustainable waste management

The local context for the UN-Habitat project 'Integrated solid waste management programme in Managua' is the city of Managua, the capital of Nicaragua, with about one million inhabitants, and its waste management. Approximately 1,200 metric tonnes of waste is collected daily by the local government's waste organisation. The waste in Managua is highly organic (around 70-80 per cent), much of it being plants and garden waste, which could be composted, although the composition of the waste is a bit dry to be ideal for that purpose.

Managua's waste collection fleet consists of more than 80 vehicles, around 40 of them modern compaction trucks donated by Italy in 2008; the rest of the fleet is a mixture or "salad" as one officer said (interview). About 40 per cent of Managua consists of informal settlements distinguished by narrow alleys full of potholes, a multitude of hanging cables and other hindrances to waste collection vehicles. New and technologically advanced, but delicate, waste trucks cannot enter or, if they do, will soon be ruined. Combined with the shortage of municipal resources to cover the totality of the municipality, this leaves a big part of the city out of the formal waste collecting service.

The collected waste is transported to La Chureca, Managua's city dump. In 2008 the dump slum was home for almost 300 families. Around 2,000 people worked daily by collecting, sorting and selling recyclables and valuables found among the rubbish. Women, men and children (around 600 at the latest count) still work daily in extremely unhealthy conditions, exposed to poisons and contamination. On top of that, the conditions in which the rubbish is mismanaged (or rather un-managed) at the dump are causing heavy contamination of the nearby Lake Xolotlán, and affecting the health and environmental safety not only of La Chureca's dwellers, but also of the whole metropolitan region of Managua. Both the informal settlements around the city, and the city dump, are the subject of development aid projects.

Since 2008, the Spanish Agency for International Development Cooperation (AECID) has funded the Acahualinca Development Project in partnership with the Managua local government. The project has three components: (1) an environmental component regarding the closing of the city dump, the construction of a classification platform and the formulation of a waste management strategy for the municipality of Managua; (2) a housing component to build up the houses for La Chureca's dwellers and the town planning of Acahualinca; and (3) a socioeconomic component of education, healthcare and childcare to support the local population to face a new life. When this chapter was written, the project was in its final phase, and the city dump is no longer open, but is instead a closed landfill with a recycling station.

The objective of UN-Habitat's project is 'to assist and integrate the AECID Programme through different initiatives supporting environmental, residential, economic and social development in the target sector of Acahualinca; and to improve the efficiency of the SWM [strategic waste management] system in Managua and in the region' (UN-Habitat, 2010b). The project has four components with the specific objectives as follows:

> 1. To provide direct support to the AECID Programme, with particular emphasis on the strengthening of livelihoods in the value chain of waste collection and recycling.
> 2. To improve municipal efficiency in solid waste management.
> 3. To improve public, private and social partnerships within the recycling sector, through direct support to the informal and formal waste recycling sectors.
> 4. To build regional capacity for improved solid waste management. (UN-Habitat, 2010b: 34)

The first objective, to support the AECID Project, is left out of this analysis, since it is stated in the project presentation that the other objectives have been the focus (UN-Habitat, 2010b: 34). To improve municipal efficiency (Objective 2), the focus has been on cost reduction and to provide a suitable and trustworthy service in Managua. Based on a waste study (generation, composition, density) done in January 2009, UN-Habitat supported local government to analyse the collection, transformation and disposal of the solid waste in order to produce a new, detailed plan with short, medium and long-term objectives. Apart from the work with the plan for solid waste, two main activities have been undertaken: first, a number of workshops within local government to decide on priorities for the modernisation of the vehicle fleet – what spares are needed, and how best to organise the repair and maintenance of the vehicles to get the most out of the fleet; and second, a pilot project of the construction of a waste transfer station in one of the *barrios*. In this project micro-enterprises collect the waste from the households, transport it on horse carts or bicycles to a waste transference station where the municipal trucks can collect it, and then transport the waste to the dump, thus saving the trucks from the poor quality streets and, by reducing the transport distance, using them more efficiently.

With respect to partnerships within the recycling sector (Objective 3), UN-Habitat has mapped the recycling sector in Managua to estimate its size and its turnover in order to be able to assess its potential and needs, for example, what technological investments are needed. For the fourth objective, regional capacity building, UN-Habitat has arranged workshops in Central America to establish a network where experiences and best practice can be shared between the countries in the region.

Global ideas and local practice

Table 5.1 provides an overview of the global ideas and related local practice. The discussion below focuses on the relative accord between the two levels and, based on close reading of the texts, what views and ideas on sustainable waste management are promoted and practised in Managua.

Table 5.1: Global and local ideas on city waste management

Global idea	Local practice
Different approaches to local problems	- Four objectives, four approaches, but more benchmarking than local adaption - Applying the model of waste transference stations, workshops based on earlier projects in other countries
Data is power: indicators of good practice	In the project, data is sought and produced about the waste and its collection, but not much with respect to income
Consider all dimensions of integrated, sustainable waste management	Physical side is considered as well as capacity in the *barrios*
Building recycling rates	Working with the recyclers
A focus on waste reduction	Not seen; focuses on waste separation and transportation
Use all available sources of finance	Heavily based on donations; the development of functioning systems for taxes, fees and other sources is not prominent
A sustainable local solution must be acceptable, appropriate and affordable in the local circumstances	Doubtful, but the partnerships with cooperatives for collection and the recycling enterprises might indicate a change

Source: Derived from UN-Habitat (2008, 2010a, 2010b)

Different approaches to local problems

At the global level, UN-Habitat promotes the importance of locally grounded solutions so that every city waste management system's background, design and local knowledge are identified when solutions or improvements are promoted. At the local level, waste transference stations are the solution that is, in practice, promoted by UN-Habitat in Managua, in workshops and best practice collections. Although the same solution everywhere does not leave much room for local adaption: waste transference stations might be designed differently locally, but the idea remains unchanged.

What is striking with the text is that much of the global and local contexts is left out; only waste management – or rather, waste transportation – is in focus. To start with, waste is disconnected from production and thus disembedded from its very global nature, whereby the global responsibility for waste production in the wealthy countries, and the flow of hazardous waste towards other geographies, is not problematised, nor are the global impacts of waste mismanagement and the excess of waste production.

Furthermore, the project aims to improve municipal efficiency in solid waste management; to do that 'a detailed analysis of solid waste collection, transfer and disposal' (UN-Habitat, 2010b: 34) has been undertaken in order to develop a plan, with the focus on cost reduction. Municipal efficiency, however, is a broad concept, and much more could have been analysed, for instance, with respect to how solid waste management corresponds with the rest of the municipal organisation, which therefore leads to questions about money: costs and incomes; priorities and consumption; how waste management is and should be funded, and by whom; whether waste management is organised in order to meet the priorities of local politicians; and how the production of waste can be decreased. By focusing only on the collection, transportation and disposal side of waste management and the cost side, waste is 'black-boxed' (Latour, 1987), thus radically narrowing the importance of the project.

Data is power

A key element in sustainable waste management as promoted by UN-Habitat is the power of data. As noted above, data is sought on waste (consistency) and how it is collected in Managua. If the focus was the waste management system, more sides of the system could be addressed. From a city management perspective the level of ignorance of the income side (including the accounting system, fees and investment plans) of the system is remarkable and something that has to be solved in order to break donor dependency and to build a sustainable waste management system that includes administrative as well as physical dimensions. A low-cost solution can be too high if there is no income. Having said that, it is also liberating that the project does not treat the income side as a medium for fantasies, as so often seen in city planning and visioning (Kornberger, 2012).

The preferences and views of the population of Managua on consumption, waste and waste management could also be collected and used as data in the waste management system, but they are not. Instead, focus is on the waste, its consistency and the amount, which is sufficient for the purpose of collecting, transporting and disposing of waste. As shown in Chapter Eight, this is significant for what they call a 'landfilling waste regime', where 'waste is considered something inert that should be accumulated in some (remote) place', which is what UN-Habitat seem to promote. Corvellec and Hultman (in Chapter Eight) observe a 'wasting less' regime, where 'waste is something that should not become', and call for data other than the physical features of waste; their stance is with a different moral, 'one must not produce waste', and they demand a change of the inhabitants' and other actors' behaviours.

Consider all dimensions of integrated, sustainable waste management

To consider all dimensions is an ambitious goal, especially when it is difficult to know what the dimensions are. As already noted, the local programme mainly focuses on the collection, transportation and disposal of waste. On the global level, it is stated that inclusivity, including 'both the users and the service provider' (UN-Habitat 2010a: 207), is a key element in sustainable waste management. What 'all dimensions' means is essential here. One way to understand different approaches to waste management and its objective is the European Union's (EU) waste hierarchy (European Commission, 2008), which ranks different outcomes of waste handling methods according to their environmental impact (see also Chapter Eight, this volume). Highest ranked is waste prevention; lowest ranked is landfill.

Waste prevention and landfill might both be examples of waste management methods, but they do range over different dimensions. Landfill is about collecting the waste and transporting it to the landfill site for disposal. Waste prevention is different entirely (for instance, if successful, there is no waste to collect), but waste prevention is at the other side of the product cycle of the landfill, at the production side: if less stuff is produced, less waste is produced too, which means that 'both users and service providers' (UN-Habitat, 2010a: 207) are some of the actors involved who should be included.

Managua is not part of the EU and the waste hierarchy does not apply there. When the project of improving waste management began, Managua's waste management was not even at the lowest level of the hierarchy, with its open city dump. So, to aim at waste prevention might be over the top, but then again, why not aim high? If all dimensions of ISWM are to be considered, more actors need to be addressed, and if the waste management is to be integrated, then into what?

Building recycling rates

In the texts discussed above, the possibility to recover, recycle and resell much of the waste is presented as an opportunity and a way towards sustainability. But what about the waste that cannot be recycled and sold, the 'unwanted' waste? Who is supposed to take care of it, and who will bear the costs? In a system where waste is a problem to be solved (that is, collected, transported, deposited) by local government, waste is a common bad that no one wants. When waste is defined as a commodity, a good, the question of ownership enters, who owns the waste? The solutions presented propose that micro-enterprises or cooperatives should take care of waste, sending it to waste transference stations for a fee from households. Local government would then take over the waste transference stations. This is presented as a win-win solution, where local government saves resources by not collecting waste from some parts of the spontaneous settlements, and by reducing investment to clean up illegal dumps; local collectors get a regular income and the spontaneous settlement inhabitants get a waste collection service that they did not have before. In Nicaragua, household solid waste collection is a municipal responsibility and waste is also a municipal good (or bad). So far, waste is legally considered as a common good that the local government can use to cover the costs for the system, instead of increasing taxes or fees. The more profitable the waste commodity becomes, the more intense the discussion about the ownership of and right to waste will be (see Chapter Nine, this volume), and is likely to become a debate with ideological answers.

A focus on waste reduction

A finding of the study of 20 cities' waste management systems (UN-Habitat, 2010a) was that there was a shift in focus from recycling to waste prevention. Therefore, UN-Habitat write in the global text that a key element in an ISWM approach, focusing on waste reduction, will most likely contain approaches from three directions simultaneously.

As for the first direction, from the bottom, phasing out an open dump is precisely what UN-Habitat is doing while supporting AECID in closing La Chureca. At the time of writing, the other two directions have not yet been seen in Managua, either in the project analysed here or during previous studies (see, for example, Zapata Campos and Zapata, 2012b). On the contrary, within the waste management team and the development projects about waste in Managua's staff who have been interviewed, there was a concern that the waste produced in the city consists of 60-70 per cent organic waste. Seeing waste as a resource and not as problem automatically brings the idea that low waste production is bad: if the future income for the poor is waste, more and not less waste is needed. This is quite the opposite from waste prevention.

Use all available sources of finance

The key conclusion in the global text is that a sustainable local solution must be 'acceptable, appropriate and affordable in the local circumstances', and 'one should prioritise capacity- and knowledge-building in order to develop inclusive approaches, sound institutions and proactive policies, and to work towards financial sustainability' (UN-Habitat, 2010a: 212). On the local level, the activities and the waste management system promoted by the UN-Habitat project is based on donor funding. But by letting private actors handle the recyclables, local government has lost what could possibly fund the collection and handling of non-sellable waste. Apart from donations which then leaves taxes and fees as a funding option, one might then ask why systems for fees and taxes have not been developed parallel to the improvement of waste collection and disposal. One possible answer is that there is a belief that it will be difficult to get the Managua residents to pay, and it is therefore not worth developing expensive systems that will stay unused. However, people do pay for other services (such as telephones and electricity), and therefore they may pay the waste collecting cooperatives and micro-enterprises when they collect their waste collecting fees. Another answer is that what we see is the effect of long-term dependency on non-governmental organisations (NGOs) and development aid. If much has been run as projects, managed and paid for by the NGO elite, why change? As such, the NGOs and development aid agencies weaken local government rather than strengthen it.

Conclusion

This chapter is about waste management in Nicaragua where the global North is still prevalent. The solutions to and ways to organise sustainable waste management in Managua represents what the global North considers desirable. A text is only a text. In this case, the text is solution-oriented and also summarises a project. That considered, it might be understandable that the arguments for and against the solutions have been left out, alternative solutions are not given room, and are kept hidden.

Texts do things. Their normative force has to be complied to or, if not, changed, reformulated, decoupled, circumvented, manipulated, co-opted or confronted, which in the end will take a lot of energy from the process, and influence local policy-makers. This is an example of how the concerns of the global North end up on the political agenda of the cities in the South by prioritising what aid development agencies decide are the important issues, rather than, for example, what local politicians prefer (Bachrach and Baratz, 1970). This might be good or bad, but it is an important issue to keep in mind when writing texts in a globally normative organisation.

The two texts explored here show differences: the global is more thorough and more hopeful as it can be lifted above the particulars, challenges and complexity of the specific case, and aim higher than might be possible at the local level. The texts also consist of various narratives on waste management: waste as a municipal critical service that needs to be optimised and decentralised; waste as a commodity; waste as an environmental and health problem; or waste as an opportunity. It is difficult to be consistent, but the incoherence creates contradictions such as the one between the demand for more waste (when seen as a commodity) and the call for less waste to be produced (when seen as an environmental problem). Indeed, the dichotomy between waste management and the administrative side of city management, that is, focusing on the costs and leaving out the income side, is unfortunate since it hinders the solution as being economically sustainable and probably also results in ongoing donor dependency.

The project also defines the waste management system in a way that does not include the inhabitants of Managua as co-constructors of the waste management system in their city, unlike most cities in the global North, where waste has often become invisible, black-boxed and hidden from the moment it is disposed of down the rubbish chute or from when it goes into the waste collection bin. In Managua, even wastebags are emptied and reused. Waste is visible for everybody. Waste is also visible at the illegal dumps. It is not black-boxed. The texts miss the opportunity to use the visibility of waste in Managua and its potential, for example, for promoting 'wasting less' attitudes. To make waste visible in a city in the North, many resources are needed (for example, environmental campaigns, study visits to waste infrastructures, recycling stations and incinerators). Rather than taking the opportunity for waste reduction and using the sociomateriality that the visibility of waste gives the project, it instead reiterates modernist patterns and repeats the same mistakes as the already industrialised nations by seeing waste management's main objective as ridding the city of its waste rather than preventing it.

References

Bachrach, P. and Baratz, M.S. (1970) *Power and poverty: Theory and practice*, New York: Oxford University Press.

European Commission (2008) *Directive 2008/98/EC of the European Parliament and the Council on waste and repealing certain documents*, Brussels: European Commission.

Kornberger, M. (2012) 'Governing the city. From planning to urban strategy', *Theory, Culture & Society*, vol 29, no 2, pp 84-106.

Latour, B. (1987) *Science in action: How to follow scientists and engineers through society*, Milton Keynes: Open University Press.

Martin, J. (1990) 'Deconstructing organizational taboos: The suppression of gender conflict in organizations', *Organization Science*, vol 1, no 4, pp 339-59.

Rossi, B. (2006) 'Aid policies and recipient strategies in Niger: Why donors and recipients should not be compartmentalized into separate "worlds of knowledge"', in D. Lewis and D. Mosse (eds) *Development brokers and translators: The ethnography of aid and agencies*, Bloomfield, CT: Kumarian, pp 27-49.

Sulle, A. (2010) 'The application of new public management doctrines in the developing world: an exploratory study of the autonomy and control of executive agencies in Tanzania', *Public Administration and Development*, vol 30, no 5, pp 435-54.

UN-Habitat (2008) *Medium-term strategic and institutional plan 2008-2013* (www.unhabitat.org/downloads/docs/IntroFA.pdf).

UN-Habitat (2010a) *Solid waste management in the world's cities*, London: Earthscan.

UN-Habitat (2010b) *Water sanitation for cities in Latin America and the Caribbean programme*, Nairobi: UN-Habitat.

UN-Habitat (2012) 'About us' (www.unhabitat.org/categories.asp?catid=1).

Zapata Campos, M.J. and Zapata, P. (2012a) 'Translating development aid into city management: the barrio Acahualinca integrated development programme in Managua, Nicaragua', *Public Administration and Development*, in press, DOI: 10.1002/pad.1628.

Zapata Campos, M.J. and Zapata, P. (2012b) 'Changing La Chureca. Organizing city resilience through action nets', *Journal of Change Management*, vol 12, no 3, pp 323-37.

Part III

Waste governance and management practices

SIX

Governance in a bottle

Dario Minervini

Introduction

This chapter deals with the Italian way of waste management from an empirical point of view, with the aim of showing how this policy is translated into sociotechnical practice. So, neither theoretical normative models nor a priori mechanisms of governance are verified here, but the network of formal and informal interaction is retraced, focusing on a localised and specific experience of waste management. In particular there is an attempt to analyse a specific part of Italian waste governance, consisting of a practice of glass sorting and collection, in a southern Italian city.

The practice is the starting point in retracing the complexity of such a sociotechnical phenomenon (Latour, 1992), enrolling a heterogeneous network of human and non-human entities. The analysis focuses on how municipal authorities cooperate with private waste collecting companies and on the interconnection of these actors with institutional agencies, national laws and regional rules. In this network the non-human side of governance is made up of coloured bottle banks for the urban sorted waste collection, storage areas, trucks and vans, technologies and plants as well as paper, plastic, glass, aluminium and other waste materials.

The empirical/descriptive perspective is adopted to avoid the reification of some myths of governance theorisation (as a taken-for-granted increase in democracy and participation) as the self-evident effectiveness of the market-oriented policy making inspired by new public management. At the same time this is a way of showing how Italian waste governance 'in the making' could be very different from the well known, but stereotyped, scenario characterised by a generalised institutional weakness.

To reconstruct how an embedded and empirical order (Rosenau and Cziempiel, 1992) of waste governance works in a city in southern Italy, a non-human protagonist of this field of policy, a glass bottle, is ethnographically followed from a household rubbish bin to a glass recycling centre. In what follows the main normative frames and dynamics of the Italian waste policy are quickly depicted. Then the theoretical and methodological framework about actor-network theory (ANT) and the shadowing technique, both adopted in the ethnography of the bottle, are presented. After that the presentation of the fieldwork details precedes an in-depth description of governance practices. The ethnographic account is structured in the form of a narrative developed through the chronological sequence of actions and actors observed, zooming in and out (Czarniawska, 2004: 121) of such a multiscaled governance. Finally, some insight about action and strategies, places and levels, interest and identities of Italian waste governance (in practice) are discussed.

Snapshots of Italian waste policy

Over the last few years, the Naples waste crisis has become well known through intensive international media exposure. The scenes displayed all over the world during the worst days of the crisis, when not oversimplified, showed the distinctive Italian pluralisation of private and public actors, of institutional levels of responsibility, of organisational and technological ways of urban management connected with the waste issue.

This complex scenario is the last stage of a relatively recent history that conventionally started in 1982 with the adoption of the first law on waste management (Decree of the President of the Republic no 915/82) with which Italy acknowledged the 1975 European Council Directive (Council of the European Communities, 1975). At that time national and local waste policies were inspired by the *command and control* (government) principle until the 1990s, when the national translation and adoption of *new public management* entailed a governance system based on agreements between private and public actors sharing the same policy community (Minervini, 2010).

The next legislation (Legislative Decree nos 22/97 and 152/06) stated the need for economic valorisation regarding waste management through an integrated system of waste disposal plants and technologies. The reduction of waste production and recycling material became the priority as, most recently, the thermal energy-from-waste technology.

Nowadays all the hierarchical levels of public administration are interrelated in a complex system of governance that connects sub-national and supra-national actors. In this multilevel governance civil society, institutional agencies and enterprises create networks of mutual interdependence between market and state (van Tatenhove et al, 2000;

Lewanski and Liberatore, 2002; Pellizzoni, 2004). At the same time the tasks of environmental institutional agencies, at all the hierarchical levels of decision making, are not exclusive but strictly interrelated with the competencies of other actors. Multilevel governance connects national agencies with local institutions, with the former enacting the EU super-national directives and guidelines, and the latter defining the regional plan of waste management, the concrete modalities of waste management and waste disposal (*provincial* level), and sorted waste collection (*municipal* level).

Some Italian studies have shown the interchangeable role of the public and private responsibilities in the national system of waste management, and the relevance of localistic dynamics in the governance arrangements. The output of this scenario is an explicit trade-off between national laws and local practice, with an increasing weight of the market logic over the public sphere and authority, with the downsizing of the state role as a stakeholder among others (Citroni and Lippi 2009). Moreover, the formal (legal) structure of national waste governance hides the empirical crowded network of relations and connections that shape, in practice, waste management. If we only take into account the domestic production of waste, there is great diversity in the chain of actors and operators involved in the management process, between cities and also within the same city. For these reasons the analysis of waste governance could be enhanced by focusing on what the plurality of actors at different levels do, how they cooperate and how they connect to the general aims of the waste policy.

Ethnography of a non-human in an actor-network taking care of non-humans

Because of the aim of this chapter (the unfolding of a governance network), the distinction between theory and methodology fails. Indeed, here the governance model is not considered as a model that needs to be investigated. For this reason the theoretical arguments focus on how to know what happens in a governance process and not on what governance a priori means or what administrative equilibrium it has to be.

From different perspectives, some sociologists have put forward the 'practice turn' (Schatzki et al, 2001), shifting from the 'social in theory' to the 'social in the making', that is, in our specific case, an inquiry into how actors, organisations, institutions, municipalities, laws, technologies, places and, of course, waste, are assembled in an *action-net* (Czarniawska, 2000). In particular, ANT scholars (Callon, 1986; Latour, 1988; Law,

1992) postulate the symmetry between the human and non-human agencies. The interplay of human and non-human entities situated in time and space mutually shape identities, roles and the interests of those entities; this is why an actor is enacted in the network and, in turn, enacts the network. The concept of actant, first elaborated in the Greimas semiology and then adopted by Latour in ANT, is referred to as human or non-human entities that act in an action programme. For the sake of simplicity the word 'actor' is used as synonymous of 'actant' in this chapter.

These scholars have shown how the ethnographic method could be effective in retracing 'the society in the making'. In particular two points need to be exposed; the first is related to the subject/object of research, while the latter refers to the micro-macro issue in sociology. First, the shadowing of symmetrical fieldwork, as an observation of heterogeneous actors, has to be based on an ethical empiricism (Czarniwaska, 2007: 9), that is, humans and non-humans are equally subjects of research from which the researcher gets to know specific and situated practices. Objects co-evolve with the social because they work everyday and everywhere with humans. So the researcher has to face uses, meanings and definitions of utility and adequacy emerging from a constant negotiation between humans and non-humans. Second, shadowing is a direct, participant and dynamic observation with which researchers follow the actions of a subject of research, crossing individual dynamics in organisational or institutional contexts. For this reason the tracing of the interactions is made by moving beyond the classical sociological micro/macro dichotomy; rather the researcher follows how aggregates of actors interplay in structuring the stability and irreversibility of certain networks (or better, *black boxes*). As the micro/macro is crossed and permanently recombined in ANT (Latour and Callon, 1981), so the relations could be studied along the global, regional and local scaling in a multiscaled perspective (Fagan, 2003).

Therefore, and in consideration of the above premises, it seems that non-humans, as waste or a specific waste material, could be followed through the shadowing method (Bruni, 2005). The ethnography presented in this chapter regards a non-human actor, a glass bottle, as the relational materialism (Law, 1992) of the waste multilevel and multisectoral governance. In practice, governance means a process of enrolling social organisations as municipal authorities, private companies and institutional agencies, while the non-human side is made up of storage areas, waste automatic collectors, waste compactors and trucks as well as waste materials.

Non-humans express their identities enacting their own agency in specific networks in which they are represented by the *spokespeople* (Latour, 1996) they are connected to. So non-humans are enrolled in a trial of strength finalised to a collective *action programme* (Akrich and Latour, 1992) as a policy goal, as the maximisation of the sorted waste collection and recycling.

At the same time, governance aims could not be effective if the goals of each actor and their tasks are not constantly negotiated, mutually adjusted and well recognised, or in other terms, translated and converged in obligatory passage points (Callon, 1986) that allow a flexible and dynamic durability to a policy network. The role of mediators (Latour, 2005) is fundamental in this process of assemblage, because they enact the translation of meanings and interests, assuring solidarity in the actor-network and empowering the action programme.

In the following there is an attempt to organise the fieldwork in a narrative about the dynamics of the actor-network crossed during the shadowing of the bottle along the collecting, transporting, cleaning, sorting and processing stages (see also research on the agency of a plastic bottle of water in the co-construction of social and political issues by Hawkins, 2009).

Research setting and techniques

Research was conducted in July and August 2011. The main place attended during this period, as the starting point of the shadowing, was Molfetta, a city in southern Italy in the province of Bari, with a population of 60,000. An important detail of the research is that Molfetta is the city where the author lives three days a week with his family, and so the shadowing starts from his home. So although he could be considered a 'native' in terms of citizenship, he is also a sociologist in local waste governance.

There were two main reasons for this choice. The first is that Molfetta represents a good scenario for a 'governance in practice' ethnographic observation because of the presence of one of the few urban waste selection platforms (where waste is stored and selected) in the Apulia region, and because it has an urban sorted waste collection system. The latter is related to the good conditions of access to the field facilitated by the general director of the selection platform, an engineer with longstanding and acknowledged experience, who immediately showed interest in the aims of the research and intellectual curiosity about the shadowing activities.

The object followed during the ethnography changed its shape several times – the author had to shadow a wine bottle, a pile of dirty and impure broken glass, a pile of pre-cleaned broken glass and finally, a pile of glass that was subsequently crushed and processed. In its changing shape, the bottle was physically and virtually connected with a great number of actors. And during participant observation the author used different research strategies and techniques to register and collect qualitative data coming from the different people encountered. Audio-recording was often allowed for the whole time the author was with other people while shadowing the bottle, so non-human sounds and noises such as human conversation, shouting or laughing, or just minutes of silence, were also recorded.

The shadowing, and the related ethnographic interviews, was the core of the research. And during those days the author was away from the place of observation, talking to waste management experts, sometimes interviewing them on specific issues, sometimes simply talking to them. Gathering clear field notes was one of the most important activities and, when possible, the author took pictures of the various situations and contexts faced, following the bottle. However, strategies and tricks (Becker, 1998) would not have been effective in the absence of the support of an environmental engineer. He was the gatekeeper (Garfinkel, 1967) who permitted entrance into the field, giving awareness and information and liaising with the 'native' actors.

In the following multilayered narrative, which is provided in the first person, the bottle story is mixed with normative remarking and generalisation arguments about waste governance dynamics. In order to help the reader the text indicates the story 'in practice' (P) and the normative/formal layer (F), while also referring to generalising (G). All the names reported in the ethnographic account are, of course, fictitious.

Before starting with the narrative account of waste governance in practice, the author would like to present the main character of the story, a glass bottle of red Italian wine, Chianti to be precise, or better, this was its identity before dinner with the author's family on a hot summer evening.

As the bottle lost its own use and exchange value

(P) As usual, after having a meal, the tacit division of labour between my wife and I established that I had to separate the waste materials into different coloured bins. It was a Monday evening and I knew that the next day the operators of ASM (Azienda Servizi Municipalizzati [municipal company of urban waste management and local transport]) would have passed in my street to collect the glass from the blue glass bank.

(F) Actually the research started a week before with the negotiation of field access with the General Director of ASM and after frequent conversations with the gatekeeper. The conversations were about the local waste management and organisation 'in theory' as expected by national and regional laws, contracts and formal regulations. In those situations I knew the formal identity of my wine bottle after dinner when associated with the glass bin in my kitchen. It became, in the eyes of national law, a 'substance or object whose holder discards or chooses or is obliged to discard' (Legislative Decree no 152/06), that is, waste. At this point, the bottle discarded in the bin, in Marxist words, loses its use and exchange value because in that situation it could never be associated with someone who would pay for or use it again.

(P) So the next morning I threw the wine bottle into the glass bank near my house and I did the same with the other materials I had separately collected the day before.

Figure 6.1: The bottle losing its identity

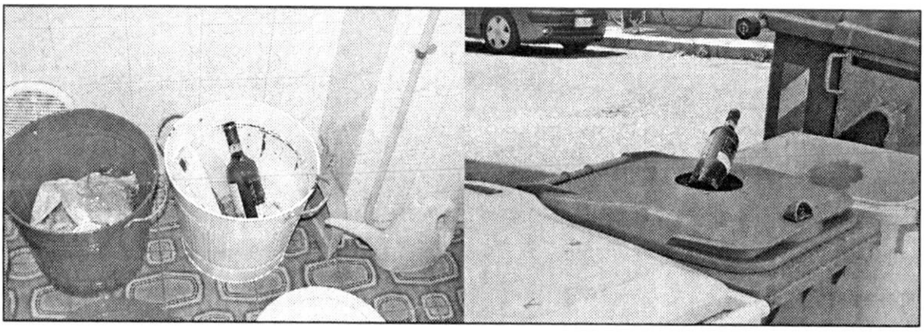

(P) Then, as agreed with the General Director, I went to the ASM buildings and waited for half an hour. In this time I observed, near the entrance of the plant, an unexpected clean and not so bad-smelling place, characterised by a precise and 'industrial' order. There was no trace of waste on the ground, and I only saw big plastic and paper bales in the middle of a regular traffic of forklifts, industrial loaders and other machines.

(F) When I was introduced to the General Director and his staff an intense conversation about the aims of the research gave a lot of relevant information about local waste governance. First it was immediately clear that the national norms, in the contexts in which I was getting my ethnography, were only the general frames of a complicated and articulated system of tasks distributed between local public and private actors:

> 'National norm established the flow of waste, from the cities to the disposal[...]. But every municipality adopts regulation strictly embedded in the local context, for example, in matters of times and frequency of collection. Thus there are different local practices of waste management and different agreements between the municipality and the private company executing collection and transport of the solid urban waste.' (ASM General Director)

The account of the General Director and his colleagues was mainly focused on the theme of the spatial organisation of waste management at sub-regional level. They confirmed what the gatekeeper told me before the shadowing started, and what the regional official documents reported about implementation in the Apulia region of the national territorial rationalisation policy of waste management through intermunicipal optimal territorial areas (*ambito territoriale ottimale*, ATO) (data and information are collected by the Ecology Department of the Apulia region and can be visited at www.rifiutiebonifica.puglia.it). In 2006 the regional authority sub-divided the territory into 15 ATOs on the basis of physical, demographic and technical parameters, with the aim of enacting integrated waste management at a sub-regional level. The ASM plant therefore became a reference point for some of the nine municipalities of the ATO named Ba1, including Molfetta.

More recently, local governance has started to be reshaped by an interesting cooperative action of four municipalities in the south of ATO Ba1 (Molfetta, Corato, Terlizzi and Bisceglie) with the aim of constituting an optimal collection area (*ambito di raccolta ottimale*, ARO). This cooperative strategy is being carried out autonomously, even if in respect of the regional guidelines on waste governance, by municipalities, the will of which is to hold the public management of the collect and transport services.

Figure 6.2: Map: spaces of governance

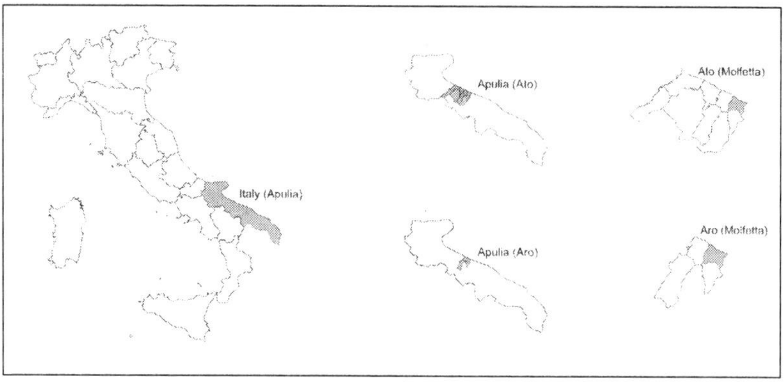

When the conversation returned to glass, the ASM General Director set out some possible scenarios:

> 'ASM consists of two sectors, the external services and the plant selection activity. As external services, we manage the collection and the transport of sorted and unsorted waste, as the street cleaning service. Glass can arrive from all three services.... The glass in the unsorted waste goes to the landfill and stays there for the next 4,000 years.... The street cleaning is a transversal service because if a roadsweeper finds a bottle, in the majority of cases he throws it in the nearest dedicated bank. When we find huge quantities of bottles in the street, for example during the Madonna dei Martiri festival [the Madonna is the patron of Molfetta and represents, with the Easter processions, the biggest religious event of the city; the festival is held for three days in September and attracts people from the surrounding cities and from all over the world], we reorganise the collection ... but it is the quantity that justifies this effort. Now we are only talking about maybe 1% of the 800 tonnes of glass we collect each year in the city.' (ASM General Director)

(P) Then someone knocked on the door. The General Director allowed the person to enter his office and introduced me to the operator I was to go with for the Tuesday route of glass collection. A few minutes later I was in a white ASM van dedicated to glass collection and transport.

As situated practices made effective (a part of) waste governance

> 'Today is a lucky day for you. You stumble on a perfect route because he [the operator indicates a van behind us] will follow us with another van for washing the banks I will empty. Antò [addressing the operator who is following], let's go to the fire brigade station.'

These were the first words of a conversation with the operator. The van I was in was one of three different vehicles ASM uses to collect glass. The other two trucks are used mainly during the night, one for the underground banks placed in the tourist area of the city, and the other for the bigger green banks placed in larger streets. The work process I observed is the most relevant in terms of quantity of glass collected, because blue glass banks are spread throughout the city.

"I have to empty more or less 150 banks, so if you want you can remain seated in the van while I'm working." These were his words when we stopped near the first glass bank.

The work was organised with a daily planning of routes covering the whole city. The day before, the same operator with the same van had done the 'commercial route', collecting glass produced during the weekend by pizzerias, bars, and so on, arriving in the extra-urban areas of the city where most of these businesses are located.

Talking about the so-called 'street route' of the other day, the operator referred to an ongoing organisation to rationalise the sub-division of the territory to cover each day. The operator's arguments about the organisation of the routes were very interesting when he showed the plans, with his personal translation of some of the places and the streets reported:

> 'Look over there [indicating the dashboard of the van], don't worry, you can do it. There are the plans of every single day, sometimes I forget the streets.... You can see my notes I signed quickly ... for some people I used their nickname. For example here it is written "household", when I read it for the first time I said: Who is "household"? After a while I understood she was the famous Lillina.'

(G) So formal documents were, using an ANT concept, translated into a full social map in which the most well known nicknames of the business owners were reported as well as the first names of the operator's relatives. But this was only one of the clever devices invented day-by-day to optimise the work, and of course, the practice of glass collection. For example, the washing van operator started his route with a clean bank attached to the back of his van. He immediately replaced the dirty bank, which had just been emptied by the other operator, and washed it while the van was travelling to the next stop. This cooperative strategy allowed just a few minutes to empty the bank, enough time for an espresso. Other expedients are depicted in the following field notes:

> 'I have to hit the brake a little bit, hold on. [the operator brakes and I hear the sound of breaking glasses coming from the tipper behind me] It's a system of mine to overfill the tipper so I don't have to return to the plant too many times ... the person who did this job before me was holding this key in his hand [the operator showed me the key he uses to open the banks before emptying them] ... I don't really know how he did it! Talking to myself I said: I have to find a solution, I should attach it like I would a dog lead.' [the operator proudly shows me the key tied with a string to a loop of his trousers]

(G) Practical experience and mental flexibility seemed the main resources of the operator to increase the effectiveness of his actions. Sometimes he adapted the route to the specific conditions he was encountering, diverting the road of the plan and emptying more banks than scheduled. And the glass collection in particular cases was informally agreed with some people who had specific needs. This was the case with some workers from the local fruit and vegetable market who usually drank beer and other beverages. If the glass bank was completely full, they took it out after the market closing, so that the operators could see it the next morning.

When we arrived where I had thrown my bottle, the operator showed me the bottle, opening the bank with his 'dog key'.

(G) All the above-mentioned actions were direct in producing an effective "association" in order to connect this glass to the whole process of valorisation of the materials collected. The operator, with his strategies and care, was, in practice, one of the main *spokespeople* of the bottle, showing what needed to be valorised, and changing the identity of the 'object whose holder had discarded it'.

Figure 6.3: The 'dog key' in action

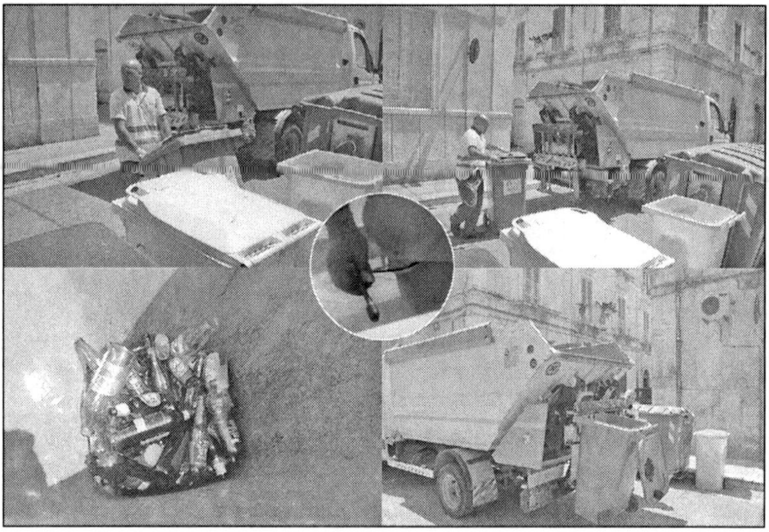

The first part of the route finished when, after the usual hit of the brakes, it was clear that the tipper was quite full. We arrived at the plant and the van with my bottle stopped on the ground scales. An employee registered the weight of the van, than the operator moved to the 'dirty glass storage area' and tipped up the glass. My wine bottle was in the middle of a lot of glass; I tried to find it, but all that I could see was what the wall inscription reported clearly: 'dirty glass' (mostly smashed).

The operator moved the van to the ground scales, again registering the weight. The results indicated that we had collected 20 quintals of glass (2,000kg), a good performance. We then completed the route with the same practices and routines, covering the remaining urban area and completing the working time of six hours.

(G) The words 'collecting' and 'transporting' provided in the official documents on actors' tasks and duties involved in the waste management were 'translated in practice' by the connection in action between the operator, his van, the 'dog key', the full social plans in which 'nice' and well-known nicknames were pinned, and the glass.

(F) Afterwards, this assemblage of practice was synthesised in a number, the weight of the glass collected, and connected by the employee of the ASM logistics office with the virtual spaces of waste governance. Indeed, municipalities, or dealers such as ASM, have to transmit the data recorded each month to the Regional Ecology Authority where other employees update the web portal on regional waste statistics. So the practice, the actors and the bottle I had followed co-constructed a number: 108,080 tonnes of glass collected for the month of July. This is only the first part of a chain of data sharing and connections that allow the Regional Agency for Environmental Prevention and Protection (Agenzia Regionale per la Prevenzione e la Protezione Ambientale, ARPA) and the Institute for Environmental Protection and Research (Istituto Superiore per la Protezione e la Ricerca Ambientale, ISPRA) to produce their annual report on the state of environmental health.

As the bottle changed shape: dimension and governance connections

The ASM logistics department is the best place to understand the glass flows and the potential governance connections that will be enacted. When I was there to understand what would happen to my bottle, I became aware that it was dispersed in the middle of a huge glass pile with bottles, pots and other glass waste objects coming from Molfetta, and also from the municipalities of Giovinazzo, Bitonto, Ruvo, Bisceglie and Corato. This meant that the subject I was following had changed its shape, its dimension and was in a wider actor-network co-constructed, until then, by several other actors I had never seen in my research activities – the public and private companies of waste collection and transport of the municipalities listed above. Indeed, these connections were extended beyond the ATO border, including Bitonto and Giovinazzo, and this was possible because of the action of another governance actor, the Italian Glass Recycle Consortium (Consorzio Recupero Vetro, CoReVe), belonging to the National Packaging Consortium (Consorzio Nazionale Imballaggi, CoNaI), one of the largest in Europe. The Consortium was created in 1997 by law (Legislative Decree no 22/97) as a non-profit organisation, even though the members are all private companies of the glass industry. Starting from 2003 the Consortium joined forces with the National Association of the Italian Municipalities (Associazione Nazionale Comuni Italiani, ANCI), and signed an agreement for transferring the funds coming from packaging (the tax of which is paid by manufacturing industries), through a system of public–private cooperation, to the municipalities engaged in the sorted waste collection. So it was thanks to the CoReVe action that the wine bottle I was shadowing was associated with glass coming from an extra ATO municipality, such as Bitonto.

(P) The day after the glass collection observation, early in the morning I was near the pile amassed in the so-called 'dirty glass storage area' of the ASM plant. After a while two operators started the process of cleaning. The first drove a yellow industrial loader, moving the glass from the 'dirty glass storage area' next to the clean area, and scattered it on the ground. Then the second, standing on a sort of carpet of broken glass, made a selection of the materials using a rake, and separated the glass from plastic shopping bags, aluminium caps and plastic. The operator searched for ceramic fragments in particular that, as he explained to me, was a serious problem for the next processing phase of glass recycling because of the different fusion temperature. After that the loader driver compacted the clean pile and repeated the process just described, emptying the 'dirty glass storage area'.

Figure 6.4: New glass size, shape and quality

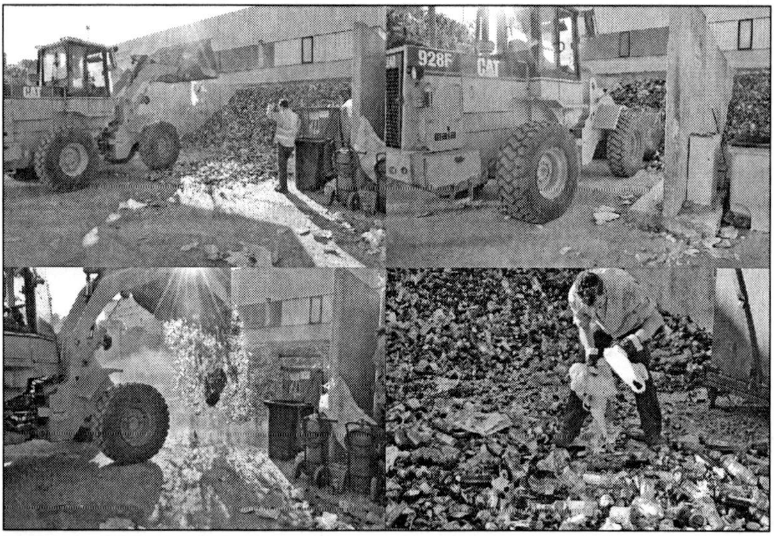

(F) This process changed the quality and quantity of the new (collective) object I had to follow. The wine bottle was still part of a pile of waste, but labelled by the governance actors as 'pre-selected'. The passage from dirty to clean status coincided in practice with the elimination of 3 per cent of impurities. This percentage was controlled and attested with unexpected rounds by CoReVe officials who assigned a quality level to the pre-selected glass, so that plant employees had to carefully verify the content of the trucks arriving in the plant, in particular those coming from other cities that may adopt other collection systems. Sometimes the entry controls of the ASM operators ended with refusal to accept the glass collected and transported for pre-selection. Thanks to this attention, the quality level certified by CoReVe for ASM was the highest at the time of the research.

The acronym CoReVe was repeated several times in the arguments of the logistics department employee, and also when he illustrated the possible scenarios after the pre-selection operation:

> 'When the municipalities have an agreement with CoReVe we have to deliver their clean glass to the destiny indicated by the consortium. The Glass of Bitonto has to go to a plant in Trani. We cannot deliver it to anybody else.... Otherwise when the municipality we furnish the service for doesn't have an agreement with CoReVe we can fix the destiny searching the best market supply.' (ASM logistics employee)

(G) Another recurrent word at this stage of the research was 'destiny' (more in ANT style than destination), which the employees called the private companies where the glass was directed for the processing phase. The destiny of the majority of glass collected and stored in the ASM plant was in the hands of CoReVe (and, of course, CoNaI), a hybrid actor conceived by the state for the public interest and enacted by private companies active in the market. This was one of the most interesting mediators of the entire governance action-net. Such a mediator shifts the local action of glass collecting, transporting and processing on the national level. In doing so, it co-produced the next step in the wine bottle journey, because the municipality of Molfetta was in agreement with CoReVe that identified the private company Recycling Glass Centre (Centro Raccolta Vetro, CRV) in the nearby city of Trani as the destiny of the glass collected and pre-selected by ASM.

But the CoReVe assemblage was not the only destiny of the clean glass stored in ASM. Only one day before my bottle had arrived at ASM, a glass load departed from there and went to a plant near Modena, in the north of Italy. This destiny, called 'extra-agreement', was negotiated directly by ASM officials, a destiny far away, that fortunately, I did not have to follow.

As the glass got a new use and exchange value

(P) Generally the clear glass pile leaves the plant for its destiny only when it reaches a significant quantity to justify the transport, which is, more or less, 30 tonnes. I had to wait 10 days before I received an email by the ASM technical department chief with the details of the next stage. So I followed the clean glass loaded on a truck and transported to another plant. When we arrived at CoReVe in Trani, I met one of the owners of the CRV plant, a company with a long story.

> 'My grandfather did this work. He did it in a rudimentary way, with a door-to-door collection. This happened after the Second World War, when he supervised some guys who went around knocking on doors asking for unused glass bottles.... Today the relation between workers and technologies is inverted. The adoption of technological innovation is a must in this market because of the high quality of materials demanded by the glass manufacturing companies.' (CRV owner)

The ASM truck unloaded the clean glass into storage areas and it was piled up on top of other glass coming from all over the centre and south of Italy. The quantity of material and the rapidity of the industrial process was very impressive: about 30 trucks a week and about 900 tonnes of glass processed 'last in last out'. As the owner confirmed, the collection of large pre-selected glass quantities was the only way to make a profit in a public–private market consisting of powerful actors such as CoReVe and multinational manufacturing companies.

The glass I was shadowing was no more a CoReVe certified first class material (but was still waste) but the property of CRV that processed it into a new raw material adopted by a well-articulated plant. The shadowing directed me through many interconnected spaces until this stage, when the glass processing was concentrated, according to ANT scholars terms, in a black box, a closed sociotechnical assemblage, as was the CRV plant.

The clean glass that had been placed in the storage area only some minutes before was immediately loaded into a hopper, one of the few external (and visible) elements of the plant. Then, following the glass into the plant, I saw a completely automated system. This was the description of the process made by the CRV owner:

> 'Here we produce the secondary raw material [the secondary raw material coming from the glass recycling is best known as cullet in English-speaking countries.].... We have powerful aspirators for the light materials like paper, adhesives, plastic shoppers, corks.... [he shows me these big aspirators placed at the first part of the production line]
>
> 'Then the conveyor belt passes through a magnetic field, where metal contaminants are separated from the glass.... Instead the non-magnetic metals are expelled by using the Eddy Current principle. [I observed caps literally jumping and falling in a dedicated container]
>
> 'The next selection concerns opaque materials such as ceramic pieces and stones. They are detected with the transparency principle. They pass over optical sensors, if the rays passed through the material, it's glass, if it doesn't, an air compressed jet eliminates the opaque material.'

(G) When I was outside, at the back of the plant, I saw a pile of multicoloured tiny pieces of glass, all of the same dimension. This was the last object of my observation, a pile of new raw material. In formal terms this was a completely new status, very different from the first one of waste glass, and it implied some consequences in practice. This last passage in a new configuration enacted again the use value (as raw material) and the exchange value (at the market price) that the wine bottle had lost in my rubbish bin.

Another aspect regarded the conditions. According to the 'last in last out' CRV organisation, about 30 tonnes of this new material was loaded onto a CRV articulated truck. Now the driver did not have to take the special waste form with him that is usually used in taking ASM pre-selected glass, but simply a transport document generally used in the case of any material transport. So here ended my governance crossing observation.

The new assemblage (cullets, articulated truck, driver) left the plant for a new destiny, a furnace in Bari, part of one of the biggest multinational glass packaging companies in the world, with 81 plants in 21 countries. But this was the starting point of another story I left to the people behind me.

Figure 6.5: Arrivederci

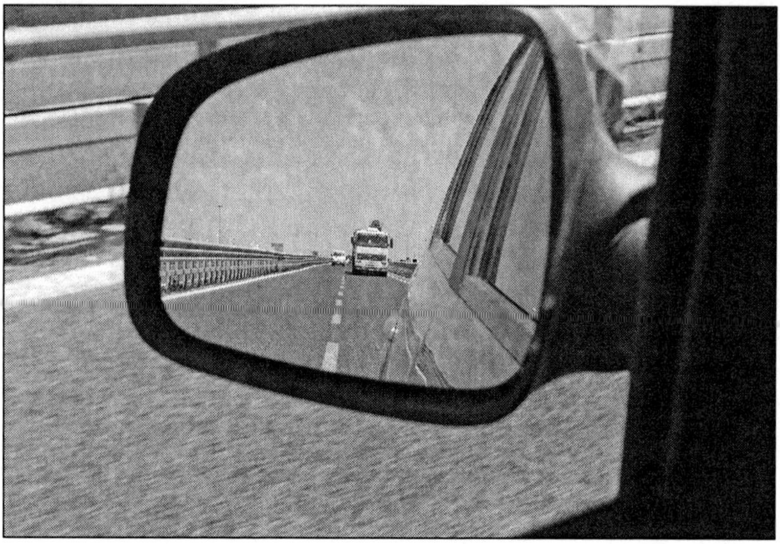

Conclusion

The shadowing of the wine bottle touched only part of the bigger action-net constituting Italian waste governance, in which everyday waste stories unfold through places and times in the national scenario. Even if embedded practices translate formal models and regulations into more or less effective synergic connections, some dynamics and aspects of the ordinary weeks of a glass wine bottle could be considered in general terms. Three main issues in particular emerge from the research: action and strategies, places and levels, and interest and identities.

First, it seems clear that a well-distributed system of competencies and tasks, established by European, national and local administrative policy makers, is unable to implement a 'one best way' of waste governance. Individual practical solutions (for example, the dog key), organisational arrangements (flexibility in the employees and the means of production) and variable geometries of governance configurations between market and state (informal agreements about tasks and needs) determine the effectiveness of waste policy. These strategies are co-constructed with the agency of objects, instruments, technologies and, of course, waste. The dog key, associated with its operator, and the blue bottle bank, sped up the emptying of the bottle banks, increasing the effectiveness of the whole process as ceramic fragments slowed down the selection and processing stage. Good or bad attachement (Latour, 1999) make the difference in the output of translation processes, that is, a high or low quantity of sorted glass, collected, transported, processed and recycled.

The second issue is about the geography of waste governance (Davies, 2008). Even if the story of the bottle that was followed took place in three neighbouring cities (Molfetta, Trani and Bari), many other spaces were virtually connected in such a multilevel governance. The case of the connection between the situated practice of waste management and the portal of the regional authority brings to light only one example of how the national level may interact with the local one. Also, in the case of the place issue, objects as materiality must be taken in a symmetric account (Law, 1999). A bottle thrown into a rubbish bin in a city in southern Italy was translated in a few weeks not only in the material output of politicians' and officials' efforts lavished in Bruxelles or Rome for a waste sustainable policy, but also in an element of profit for a big company, the headquarters of which are in the US (see also Gregson et al, 2010). This happened because a complex sociotechnical chain of actors, spokespeople, mediators and black boxes did their work effectively, constantly linking the local with the global. And this is why it could be more interesting to retrace how actors work and engage with other networks instead of explaining why macro- or micro-actors do what they do.

The third issue is strictly associated with the second, and concerns identities and interests in waste governance, recalling the theme of power. To be more precise, the inquiry is into the way power is made and co-constructed. As shown in the ethnographic account, a high number of synergies increasingly shaped the extension of the assemblage involved in governing the management of sorted waste. This process translates identities of each actor into a more coherent programme of action oriented to the economic valorisation of broken glass. This happened through the sociological classical dimensional scale, from micro to macro and vice versa, connecting in time and space individual actors or objects as organisations and technological infrastructures. In practice the assemblage increased its dimension and, of course, its influence to translate other elements in the chain. The research demonstrates the relevance of dispositive that allows translation and alignment of heterogeneous interests into points of obligatory passage and, arguably, the coordination of actions in a specific policy programme. The example of CoReVe is quite clear. This network connected with the local networks of waste management that influence most of the recycled market in Italy. The end to the shadowing shows the highest level of aggregated entities in a programme of action, with the presence of one international player completing the chain of recycling. This makes the whole programme established in multilevel governance powerful (in the sense of effective), and translated in practice by a network of actors and strategies.

As shown in the first section of this chapter, many studies have shown the weakness coming from the fragmentation and pluralisation of waste governance, from a normative and regulative point of view. Here we underline how this fragmentation exists, even if we consider the practice (and informal) side of governance, because of local informal actions, experiences, strategies and histories. The governing of waste in the cities is made of heterogeneous entities, that is, unwelcome actors as well (criminal organisations could associate or be associated with the network). At the same time, this fragmentation means a certain degree of autonomy to enhance the connection between responsibilities and competencies, and sometimes to create new embedded solutions to manage waste flow. This is why the operator hitting the brake, the ARO experiment and the other practices observed following a simple wine bottle had the power to co-construct political and ethical meanings (Hawkins, 2006) as the exchange and use value of the same bottle.

References

Akrich, M. and Latour, B. (1992) 'A summary of a convenient vocabulary for the semiotics of human and nonhuman assemblies', in W. Bijker and J. Law (1992) *Shaping technology, building society: Studies in sociotechnical change*, Cambridge, MA: The MIT Press, pp 259-64.

Becker, H.S. (1998) *Tricks of the trade: How to think about your research while you're doing it*, Chicago, IL: University of Chicago Press.

Bruni, E.A. (2005) 'Shadowing software and clinical records: On the ethnography of non-humans and heterogeneous contexts', *Organization*, vol 12, no 3, pp 357-78.

Callon, M. (1986) 'Some elements of a sociology of translation: Domestication of the scallops and the fishermen of St Brieuc Bay', in J. Law (ed) *Power, action and belief: A new sociology of knowledge*, London: Routledge & Kegan Paul, pp 196-233.

Callon, M. and Latour, B. (1981) 'Unscrewing the big leviathan: How actors macro-structure reality and how sociologist help them to do so', in K. Knorr-Cetina and A.V. Cicouvel (eds) *Advances in social theory and methodology: Towards an integration of micro and macro-sociology*, London: Routledge, pp 277-303.

Citroni, G. and Lippi, A. (2009) 'Pubblico e privato nella governance dei rifiuti in Italia', *Rivista Italiana di politiche pubbliche*, no 1, pp 71-108.

Council of the European Communities (1975) *Council Directive 75/442/EEC of 15 July 1975 on waste*, Brussels: Council of the European Communities.

Czarniawska, B. (2000) *A city reframed: Managing Warsaw in the 1990s*, Amsterdam: Harwood Academic Publishers.

Czarniawska, B. (2004) *Narratives in social science research: Introducing qualitative methods*, London: Sage Publications.

Czarniawska, B. (2007) *Shadowing: And other techniques for doing fieldwork in modern societies*, Copenhagen: Copenhagen Business School Press.

Davies, A.R. (2008) *The geographies of garbage governance: Interventions, interactions, and outcomes*, Aldershot: Ashgate.

Fagan, H. (2003) 'Sociological reflections on governing waste', *Irish Journal of Sociology*, vol 12, no 1, pp 67-85.

Garfinkel, H. (1967) *Studies in ethnomethodology*, Englewood Cliffs, NJ: Prentice-Hall.

Gregson, N., Crang, M., Ahamed, F., Akhtar, N. and Ferdous, R. (2010) 'Following things of rubbish value: end-of-life ships, "chock-chocky" furniture and the Bangladeshi middle class consumer', *Geoforum*, vol 41, no 6, pp 846-54.

Hawkins, G. (2006) *The ethics of waste: How we relate to rubbish*, Lanham, MD: Rowman & Littlefield.

Hawkins, G. (2009) 'The politics of bottled water: Assembling bottled water as brand, waste and oil', *Journal of Cultural Economy*, vol 2, nos 1/2, pp 183-95.

Law, J. (1992) 'Notes on the theory of the actor network: Ordering, strategy and heterogeneity', *Systems Practice*, vol 5, no 4, pp 379-93.

Law, J. (1999) *Materialities, spatialities, globalities*, Lancaster: Centre for Science Studies, Lancaster University.

Latour, B. (1988) 'Mixing humans and nonhumans together: The sociology of a door-closer', *Social Problems*, vol 35, no 3, pp 298-310.

Latour, B. (1992) 'Where are the missing masses? Sociology of a few mundane artefacts', in W. Bijker and J. Law (eds) *Shaping technology, building society: Studies in sociotechnical change*, Cambridge, MA: The MIT Press, pp 225-58.

Latour, B. (1996) *Aramis, or the Love of technology*. Cambridge, MA: The MIT Press.

Latour, B. (1999) *Politiques de la nature*, Paris: La découverte.

Lewanski, R. and Liberatore, A. (2002) 'Environment protection in Italy. Analyzing the local, national and EC level of policy making', in U. Desai *Environmental politics and policy in industrialized countries*, Cambridge, MA: The MIT Press, pp 203-47.

Minervini, D. (2010) *Politica e rifiuti*, Napoli: Liguori.

Pellizzoni, L. (2004) 'Responsibility and environmental governance', *Environmental Politics*, vol.13, no 3, pp 541-65.

Rosenau, J.N. and Czempiel, E.O. (eds) (1992) *Governance without government: Order and change in world politics*, Cambridge: Cambridge University Press.

Schatzki, T.R., Knorr Cetina, K. and von Savigny, E. (eds) (2001) *The practice turn in contemporary theory*, London: Routledge.

van Tatenhove, J., Arts, B. and Leroy, P. (eds) (2000) *Political modernisation and the environment: The renewal of environmental policy arrangements*. Dordrecht: Kluwer Academic Publishers.

SEVEN

Hybrid organisations in waste management: public and private organisations in a deregulated market environment

Philip Marcel Karré

Introduction

The state and the market are two distinct sectors: whereas the state (or public sector) looks out for the common good, the market's (or private sector's) main objective is to realise a profit. Both sectors have their own set of rules, norms and values, and thus very distinct cultures. Waste management operates in the border area of these two sectors. This holds true for both the supply and the demand side: we see both public and private *customers* (in many countries, collecting and disposing of household waste is a statutory task of [local] governments, while for businesses, disposing of waste is often their own responsibility) and both public and private *providers*. This creates a mixed market in which both state-owned and commercial organisations operate, each with their own private business interests.

But also within these organisations themselves, this mixing takes place: public (that is, state-owned) waste management services are now often run as if they were commercial companies, and also engage in the collection and disposal of business waste, a market segment which, until very recently, was the domain of their private rivals. And these commercial, often multinational and stock exchange listed, enterprises have become active in the market for the collection and disposal of household waste. As a result, waste management has become a mix of public and private, and hence a hybrid activity undertaken by hybrid organisations.

This chapter examines this hybridity in waste management. It discusses what it means, how it manifests itself and what opportunities and dilemmas it raises. It does this by taking the Dutch waste management sector as an example, which over the last two decades has developed into a highly dynamic and hybrid marketplace in which many hybrid waste management organisations operate. As such it can serve as an ideal illustration of the changes the waste management sectors of many other countries have undergone. The chapter first refines the definition of hybridity by identifying the public and private interests that come together in hybrid organisations in the waste management sector. It illustrates this by looking at the example of the Netherlands, and not only describes what types of hybrid organisations can be found there, but also which issues arise due to their hybrid status in relationship with their political overlords, competitors and employees and citizens. It concludes with a discussion of the hybrid nature of many waste management organisations and the questions it raises.

Public and private interests in waste management

Waste management is big business. In 2008, the three biggest players in the European market (French Veolia and Suez Environnement, and German REMONDIS) shared sales of €20 billion (Hall, 2010). But waste is not only a business. Waste management organisations also fulfil important tasks for society, as their services bear a direct connection to the state of our economy and our quality of life. This becomes painfully obvious when waste management suddenly stops, which can happen as a result of labour disputes and strikes. Notably, such episodes occurred during Britain's Winter of Discontent in 1978/79 and, more recently, in the Italian city of Naples, in 2008.

It is to everyone's advantage that waste is properly taken care of; after all, no one wants rubbish piled high on the streets, not just because of the unpleasant sights and smells, but also because of the health hazard it would cause, the pests it would attract, and the potential pollution of drinking water. Because public interest is at stake in waste management, governments traditionally play an important role in the collection and disposal of waste in many countries around the world. In the past, many chose to provide waste management services themselves, by establishing their own collection services and building their own waste disposal plants.

Good waste management is in the public interest for several reasons. For example, the Dutch government lists the following (Afval Overleg Orgaan, 2002, based on Ministerie van Economische Zaken, 2000):

- *Universal provision:* waste management is generally considered to be an essential service to society for the reasons mentioned before.

Therefore it is considered desirable that everybody should have access to waste management services on a non-discriminatory basis, and under transparent conditions. The prices for the collection and disposal of waste are expected to be directly related to the costs of services delivered.

- *Continuity of sufficient capacity:* there will always be waste that cannot be recycled and therefore has to be either disposed of at landfills or has to be incinerated. It is in the public's interest that a sufficient amount of landfill and incineration capacity is available, and that the continuity of these installations is guaranteed.
- *Protection of captive customers:* there are captive customers in waste management. For example, individual households generally cannot choose the company that empties their bins; government makes that decision for them. Hence there is, at least from the point of view of the individual citizen, no real market for waste. It is in the public interest to protect captive customers from paying too much for the provision of waste services.
- *Environmental, public safety and health concerns:* proper waste management has a positive effect on the environment, public safety and health. Government is therefore expected to employ an active waste management policy to guarantee this.
- *Efficient markets and functional regulation:* waste management takes place in a regulated environment. Due to the environmental, public safety and health concerns mentioned before it is not in the public interest to totally liberalise this market. There will always be a task for government, for example, in making regulations about the type and technical specifications of waste management installations that are allowed to be built and by controlling prices, for example, by levying taxes for certain services such as landfilling.

Since the 1990s broader political developments have changed governments' roles in waste management. In a liberalisation (or better, deregulation, as some rules still stay in place) of the waste management sector, many governments have chosen to switch from *providing* to *ensuring* this public service by contracting out its provision to private companies or to government-owned waste management organisations which, following the principles of New Public Management, were transformed to be run along more business-like lines (cf Greve, 2007; Skelcher, 2007; Christensen and Lægreid, 2011; Pollitt and Bouckaert, 2011). As a result, there is now a wide array of hybrid organisations in this sector, which can be defined as 'heterogeneous arrangements, characterised by mixtures of pure and incongruous origins, (ideal) types, "cultures", "coordination mechanisms", "rationalities", or "action logics"' (Brandsen et al, 2005: 750).

These hybrid waste organisations collect or dispose of municipal *and* industrial waste and receive public *and* private funding and incentives. They *mix* public with private business interests, steering mechanisms and governance arrangements. This inevitably leads to tensions. For example, while it can be in the public interest that those living in remote areas should have access to affordable waste management services, providing them at such rates can run contrary to a company's interest of making a profit.

Another example of tensions due to hybridity, at least according to their private rivals, is that public waste management organisations that also collect business waste distort free competition as they can use public funds to compete. This is unfair to both their private rivals who do not have access to these vast levels of interest-free cash, but also, these rivals claim, to taxpayers, since their money is improperly used for inherently risky business ventures. Because these organisations often operate at arm's length of government as a result of New Public Management reforms, there is a possible lack of democratic control that could prevent a loss of public funds.

But hybridity does not necessarily have only detrimental effects. The tensions that arise through bringing public and private together can also be beneficial. Embracing a more business-like manner of work can increase the quality of the service provision of public waste management organisations through a focus on more efficiency and effectiveness. Public waste management organisations can also use profits they generate on the commercial waste management market to subsidise their public service provision. An increased orientation on the customers of waste collection and disposal, as opposed to a focus on government as a subsidiser, can also be a powerful incentive for an organisation to be more open and transparent in its governance and accountability arrangements.

To summarise, within waste management public and private come together in various ways. Waste management is inherently hybrid, as by definition it mixes public and private interests. Due to the liberalisation/deregulation of the waste market and New Public Management-styled reforms of many public waste management organisations, increasing numbers of hybrid organisations have emerged that now also have to mix public and private within themselves.

Their hybridity can produce positive and negative economic, performance-related, cultural and governance-related effects (for an overview of the literature on which these effects are based, see chapter 3 in Karré, 2011). The first deals with the impact it has on free competition and the financial performance of an organisation; the second with the impact it has on the quality of its service provision; the third deals with its impact on an organisation's culture; and the last, with its accountability towards, and supervision from, its political principals. Based on this, we can state that hybridity has an influence on several of the organisation's relationships with internal and external parties: economic effects mostly influence an organisation's relationship with its commercial rivals; performance-related effects influence the relationships with citizens; cultural effects influence the relationship between an organisation's management and staff; and governance-related effects influence the relationship an organisation has with its political overlords.

This chapter takes a closer look at the positive and negative effects caused by hybridity by examining how they manifest themselves in waste management in the Netherlands. First, however, we describe the policy shifts, which turned Dutch waste management from a highly regulated sector into a hybrid marketplace, and the hybrid organisations that can be found in the market segments for the collection of household waste, the collection of business waste and the disposal of both.

Developments in the Dutch waste management sector

Policy shifts

Until the late 1990s the Dutch waste management sector was heavily regulated. Regional government monopolies dominated waste collection and waste disposal, aiming at regional self-sufficiency. This meant that until 2000 it was illegal to transport waste across provincial borders. Waste was predominantly collected by government-owned collection services, which had to dispose of it at landfills or at incineration plants within each province.

In the Dutch version of the waste hierarchy, prevention is the most desirable option, followed by recycling, then incineration, with landfilling as the last resort. Either regional or municipal governments owned all of the incineration plants and most landfilling facilities at that time. Their capacity was planned centrally, by a *Waste Management Council*, which was made up of national, regional and local governments. Because of a moratorium (lifted in 2003) on the construction of new incineration plants, which came into effect after the dioxin scandals of the 1980s, when dioxin, an allegedly carcinogenic substance, was found to not have been sufficiently filtered from the emissions of waste incineration plants, new players were prohibited from entering this market. This lack of competition led to artificially high tariffs for the incineration of waste.

As a last resort option, landfilling was very expensive and therefore no real alternative to incineration. In 1996 landfilling combustible waste was even banned, while a special landfill tax was instated for other types of waste. This tax has been increased over the years to the highest charged in any European country (Dijkgraaf, 2004: 7). This, combined with the monopoly position of incinerators, caused tariffs for the disposal of waste to be artificially high.

Discussion about the artificially high tariffs charged for the incineration of waste led to the installation of a government commission which advised the opening of regional borders for the transport of waste in 2000, creating a national market for waste treatment (Commissie Toekomstige Organisatie Afvalverwijdering, 1996). Transport of waste across national borders was still prohibited as Dutch government aimed at creating national self-sufficiency. However, there was a loophole in this transnational transport ban. European Union (EU) regulation made it possible for Dutch waste management companies to contract foreign separation companies. Thanks to EU legislation aimed at increasing the amount of waste being reused, waste was allowed to be transported abroad as long as more than 50 per cent of it was reused at its final destination. Waste collection companies used this loophole to evade high tariffs for incineration (due to the lack of competition) and landfilling (due to the landfilling tax). Most of the waste was transported to landfilling sites in Germany, where costs were much lower.

From 1 January 2007 restrictions on the transport of non-hazardous combustible waste across national borders have been eased, although regulation has stayed in place for the landfilling of waste. The capacity of landfilling facilities is still planned centrally and there is a ban in place on the export of waste to be landfilled abroad. Still, especially compared to the situation before 1997, the Dutch waste management sector now presents itself as a fairly liberalised market, in which several kinds of hybrid organisations can be found. The Netherlands is now even a major importer of waste to be disposed of, burning waste from Italy and Germany.

Hybrid organisations in waste collection

Household waste

Under Dutch law, municipalities are obliged to *ensure* the collection of household waste. In the past many municipalities did so by providing collection services themselves, but since then some have chosen to contract these services out to public and private companies or to enter into a public private partnership with a commercial waste management company. There is now a wide array of organisations active in this sector with various forms of legal status (see Table 7.1).

Table 7.1: Types of organisations in the market for the collection of household and biodegradable waste with their market shares in 2011

Type of organisation	Municipalities (%)	Households (%)
Municipal service	16	26
Municipal service of neighbouring municipality	3	2
Local joint venture	14	11
Autonomised public company	34	36
Private sector company	30	19
Public–private partnership	3	6

Source: Derived from NL Agency (2011)

In 2011, *public sector companies* were employed by 67 per cent of Dutch municipalities. They are referred to as government dominated enterprises (indicating that the influence by governmens varies in such organisations) and come in three forms: municipal services, local joint ventures and autonomised public companies. Municipalities can also choose to use the collection services of neighbouring communities.

Municipal services were employed by 16 per cent of all Dutch municipalities (among them the country's three biggest cities, Amsterdam, Rotterdam and The Hague, which meant that this group represents 26 per cent of Dutch households) in 2011. Some of them were integral parts of the municipality's hierarchy. Others were internally autonomised using a management contract.

Local joint ventures were employed by 14 per cent of Dutch municipalities in 2011. These are generally smaller municipalities that group together to achieve economies of scale, and therefore only represent 11 per cent of households. There were 11 such local joint ventures in the Netherlands in 2011.

Autonomised public companies were employed by 34 per cent of Dutch municipalities in 2006. This group consists of larger companies and smaller municipal services which were autonomised as a public company. There were 24 such autonomised public companies in the Netherlands in 2011. In the 1990s many municipal waste collection services were autonomised. In the new millennium this trend has stopped. In 2005 a survey found that about 80 per cent of Dutch municipalities had no plans to change the legal status of their waste collection services (cf. SenterNovem, 2006).

Three per cent of Dutch municipalities contracted their waste collection duties out to the *service of a neighbouring municipality*. The municipal waste collection service of the Northern provincial capital of Groningen, for example, collects waste in a number of (smaller) neighbouring municipalities.

Municipalities can also choose not to have their waste collected by public, but by private sector waste management companies, either by contracting this task out to them or by forming public–private partnerships. *Private sector companies* were employed by 30 per cent of municipalities in 2011, mostly by those that were too small to make their own collection service economically viable. SITA and Van Gansewinkel were the biggest private companies collecting household waste. All in all, the municipalities employed 15 private companies for the collection of their waste. *Partnerships* between a municipality and a private company were employed by only 3 per cent of all municipalities. Examples of such constructions were HMS (Haagse Milieu Services [The Hague Environmental Services], a public–private partnership between the municipality of The Hague and Van Gansewinkel Group waste company) and CURE (Centrum Uitvoering Reinigingstaken Eindhoven en omgeving, [Centre for Waste Management Tasks Eindhoven and surroundings]), a partnership between Van Gansewinkel and the municipality of Eindhoven).

Business waste

Municipalities are not obliged to collect business waste: businesses have to take care of this themselves. Like municipalities in the collection of household waste, they can choose from an array of arrangements. They can contract out collection activities to the municipal collector operating in their area, a private collector or a public company. Private waste management companies mostly dominate this market segment, but public enterprises increasingly compete in this market.

Hybrid organisations in waste disposal

After collection, waste needs to be disposed of. In the Netherlands this is done either by incineration or by landfilling. In contrast to waste *collection*, waste *disposal* companies generally deal with both municipal and business waste. As already mentioned, landfilling is discouraged in the Netherlands by levying a high landfill tax. There are 37 landfills in the country but most waste is burned by 10 waste incineration plants owned by seven companies (SenterNovem, 2006; updated by the author). Four are owned by local and regional governments. Ownership of a fifth is shared between several local governments and a private German waste management company. The last two are commercial companies, which are, in turn, part of international conglomerates. Of these two, Afvalverwerking Rijnmond (AVR, Waste Management Service Rijnmond) (which runs waste incineration plants in Duiven and Rozenburg) is an interesting case to highlight. Established as part of the municipality of Rotterdam, AVR developed into a multinational company and was sold in 2008 by the municipality to three private equity funds (one British, one American and one Dutch). AVR then acquired and was later merged with the Van Gansewinkel Group, a private waste management company, and is now one of Europe's biggest waste companies.

Issues with hybrid organisations in waste management

As noted earlier, waste management by hybrid organisations can potentially lead to several positive and negative economic, performance-related, cultural and governance-related effects. These influence the relationship a waste management organisation has with several internal and external parties. This chapter now discusses how this happens in practice, and to which positive and negative effects it leads, again, by taking the Dutch waste management sector as an example. Based on the results of a study of hybrid organisations in this sector (Karré, 2011), the chapter discusses how their hybridity influenced their relationships with their commercial rivals, their customers and political overlords, and its effects on the relationship between the organisations' management and staff. By doing so a picture is painted of the practical issues that arise due to organisational hybridity in waste management.

Issues concerning an organisation's relationship with its competitors

Before the emergence of hybrid organisations in this sector, there was a clear division of tasks between private waste management companies and the waste management services operated by local governments. The latter dealt with household waste within their own municipality, while the former dealt with business waste and collected household waste in those municipalities which, for one reason or another, did not have their own waste services (mainly because they were too small to make such services commercially viable). This clearly laid out world was turned on its head due to the liberalisation of the waste management sector. Now companies were free to tender for contracts everywhere in the Netherlands: the waste management *sector* had become a waste management *market*. And it was not only commercial companies that participated but also municipal waste management services.

Due to the philosophy behind New Public Management, many municipalities performed a purchaser/provider split, which meant that their waste management services were put at arm's length and approached as any other company. It was no longer a matter of course that a municipality's waste management service would also be asked to fulfil this task. It now had to tender for the contract to collect household waste in its own municipality, a process in which other companies were invited to participate.

Municipal waste management organisations started to behave like businesses to be able to withstand competition from other companies. This business-like outlook, together with the necessity of substituting decreasing municipal subsidies with income from the market, made them also try to increase their market share, either by also tendering for contracts with other municipalities or by tendering for contracts for the disposal of business waste.

By doing so, hybrid waste management companies have become *competitors* of their commercial counterparts, which did not take the challenge lying down. In the Netherlands, the rise in the number of hybrid organisations providing public services and venturing out into commercial service provision has instigated a fierce discussion about the desirability of this trend (Brandsen and Karré, 2011). Also in the waste management sector, commercial companies complain that hybrid organisations are distorting free competition, as these organisations can theoretically use public money to subsidise their market activities, and they also have other competitive advantages, for example, through regulation favouring public service provision by organisations in which governments have a controlling stake, or simply because of the personal contacts representatives of these organisations have in the town hall.

There have been a small number of highly publicised scandals in the Netherlands about hybrid organisations squandering public money through risky ventures in the commercial world, but so far not in the waste management sector. In general, there seem to be sufficient checks and balances in place to prevent such incidents (as a report on the matter by the Netherlands Court of Audit, 2004, concluded). Also, what constitutes as distorting the marketplace is in the eyes of the beholder. Evidence shows that one important reason for distorting free trade can be to guarantee public interest, for example, in the case described by Karré (2011) of a Dutch municipality that invested in a brand new and exceptionally sustainable waste incineration plant which was purpose-built to burn business waste only. From the standpoint of a commercial rival this action is despicable, whereas from a public interest view, the municipality should be applauded for such an eco-friendly investment, especially in economically difficult times in which private companies are shirking from investing in new technologies. Hybridity turns municipal organisations into the rivals of commercial companies, but as long as the public benefits surpass the risks of such an endeavour, this does not seem to be such a bad thing overall. After all, the *core business* of government is to interfere in free competition, when this is considered to be in the public interest.

Issues concerning an organisation's relationship with citizens

Before they had to deal with hybridity, that is, before they were put at arm's length, municipal waste management services were an integral part of local government bureaucracy – a hierarchy with local politicians at the top. In this system, these organisations were financed by a lump sum and there was hardly any incentive to behave in a more efficient and effective manner. After all, there was no direct link between the performance of the organisations and the funding it received: even without being overly efficient or customer-friendly, the organisation was assured of its money. If anything, trying to be more efficient could work to the organisation's disadvantage: if it was found to have any of its budget left over at the end of the year, politicians might see that as a sign they could easily make do with a little less for the next year.

This changed as municipal waste management organisations were hybridised: they were now expected to behave like businesses and were financed based on performance, that is, based on the output they generated and service levels agreed on in the contracts they had signed with the municipalities. Practically, this meant that only services that had been paid for were rendered; for example, whereas before, bulky waste may have been picked up along with regular waste collection, this was now only done on particular dates, based on the contract the company had with the municipality. This allowed for a more efficient use of the organisation's resources and kept the costs for waste collection under control, which benefited the taxpayer, but also meant a decrease in the service level experienced by citizens. Due to hybridity, municipal waste management companies also began to see citizens as customers who had to be served in an efficient manner, but only for those services they had actually paid for. In the example of bulk waste collection, this had not been the case. That such waste had been collected was a customer-friendly extra activity that, under the new financial regime, cost the organisation money which it, due to the contracts it had signed, could not ask back from the municipality.

In general, research suggests, however, that hybridity has led to higher levels of efficiency in the service provision of municipal waste management companies, due to the new organisational values brought forward through New Public Management-style reforms and a change in funding (Karré, 2011). Funding on output served as an incentive not to waste money and also led to a more business-like relationship between organisations and citizens as customers of waste management. Whereas more efficiency meant that the costs for waste management, which citizens had to cover through taxes, could be kept under control, hybridity also cost them more money, as any services beyond those bought in by the municipality had to be privately paid for separately.

Issues concerning an organisation's relationship with politics

The changing relationship between the organisation and its political principals is the first and foremost change of the hybridisation process. Hybridisation is generally defined as a change in this relationship ('putting at arm's length'), and it is the political principal who starts the formal hybridisation process by redefining its relationship with the organisation.

Typically, the relationship between the political principal and the organisation *before* it becomes hybrid is a direct, hierarchical one. The political principal decides what the organisation does, how it does that, how much funds it has to do it, and by which means. In waste management, that means that the political principal has the ultimate say on not only how often waste is collected, but also who does the collecting (which staff are hired) and which tools are used (for example, which trucks are bought).

Although in most cases some of the decision-making power is transferred to the head of the waste management organisation, the ultimate say and the ultimate responsibility lies with the political principal. Arrangements are often made by which the organisation's director can make small, day-to-day purchases independently, whereas he needs the political principal's permission for larger investments. This often results in frustration at the organisation's end, because the political decision-making process can be slow, and also because of the principal's lack of expertise needed to make such decisions (resulting in putting off the decision even longer). At one case organisation featured in Karré (2011), the managing director complained that it took months for the aldermen to decide to let him order a new truck, an essential investment for any waste management company. This frustration with political inertia often became one of the reasons for putting the organisation at arm's length. The case organisations' directors in the study mentioned before all actively lobbied for this change. However, a changing relationship does not necessarily put an end to such frustrations.

Once the organisation is put at arm's length, the political principal's role splits into two distinctive components: on the one hand, they are the *commissioning body*, and on the other, the organisation's *owner or shareholder*. As the *commissioning body*, the political principal contracts the waste management organisation to collect and dispose of household waste. Agreements are made (and laid down in a contract) about price and service level, but the details of the execution are now the organisation's own responsibility. This does not necessarily make the relationship easier: since the political principal still lacks expertise (and often even more so than before, as the municipal experts on waste are now the waste management organisation's employees, rather than the municipalities), there is often poor oversight on the contract's fulfilment. The directors of the case organisations saw this as a problem rather than a welcome *carte blanche* to do as they wished, as they saw that it was in the organisation's best interests to be held to account. In some organisations, supervisory boards were set up to create a better system of checks and balances. These functioned well as long as they were staffed with experts; political appointees, on the other hand, tended to forget about the organisation's best interests, and mainly had an eye for political interest. For example, at one waste management organisation studied, members of the supervisory board tried to install a new deputy managing director, who was clearly a crony of the chair of the board.

By letting themselves be influenced by political interests, members of an organisation's supervisory board act more according to the political principal's second role, that of *shareholder*. A shareholder's main interest is getting a return on his or her investment. In one case organisation, this resulted in an annual struggle between the municipal shareholders who demanded to be paid a dividend, and the organisation's director, who wanted to use that money to make long-term investments in his company.

Issues concerning an organisation's relationship with its staff

Hybridity also implies a change in the relationship between the organisation and its staff. As employees of a municipal department, the waste management workers enjoyed the status of civil servants, which often comes with special privileges. At the same time, personnel management had little priority. If anything, the municipality often used the waste management department as an employment opportunity for people who had few chances elsewhere, or even a convenient place to park workers who were no longer wanted at other departments, but who could not be fired either.

Although being part of the municipal bureaucracy meant there were many rules, these rules were not strictly enforced in the case organisations studied. In one organisation, the staff even ran a sideline in reclaimed metal, which they sold on for their own profit. Such practices were put to an end when the organisations were hybridised: from then on, efficiency was crucial to the organisation's survival. Therefore, compliance with the rules and performance became highly important.

All case organisations cited cultural change as one of the key conditions for running their organisations like a business. The organisations' culture needed to change from bureaucratic to business-oriented. But achieving cultural change is easier said than done: those organisations that tried to force their business-like attitude on their employees in a top-down fashion failed miserably. Those that tried connecting with the staff, convincing them of the importance of change, were much more successful, although also in those cases some employees left the organisation soon after the change because they were unable to adapt to the new circumstances.

The people who left the organisation were mostly technical professionals and middle managers, who used to be the powerful ones within the organisation. Since the directors were weak at the time the waste management organisations were municipal departments, and the rest of the municipal organisation lacked expertise, the technical experts could run their section as they saw fit. After all, they were the experts. Similarly, the middle managers often ran their sections as their own personal fiefdoms. As soon as the organisations had to become more business-like, new commercially oriented staff were brought in. Now these salespeople (equipped with expensive new company cars, or so the begrudged old guard never failed to mention) were running the show, and many of the experts felt this was no longer 'their' organisation.

Hybridity changes the relationship between an organisation's management and its staff as it shifts the balance of power. Now the management becomes the dominant force within the organisation, whereas before it lay with the experts. This not only leads to a stronger focus on financial performance, but also means that compliance with organisational rules and regulations becomes more important. Those are now the rules to discipline the workforce and its behaviour.

Conclusion

This chapter has discussed the hybrid character of the waste management sector and especially the role played by hybrid organisations. Waste management has always been a hybrid activity, mixing public and private on several levels, but this is increasingly true as more and more hybrid organisations come to operate in what has become a real market. This is due to a liberalisation/deregulation of waste management, as stringent rules and regulations are relaxed to allow market mechanisms to unfold their positive effects, and because municipal waste management services have begun to behave like real companies under the influence of New Public Management. However, the change towards a market is (not yet) fully-fledged. There are many public interests at stake in waste management, making government involvement not only desirable but also necessary in preventing the negative side effects of market forces. And while many local governments have allowed their waste services to behave like companies, in many cases they have decided not to privatise them by selling them off to their private rivals. These developments make waste management even more hybrid, as public and private interests come together within organisations, forcing them to adopt new tasks, embrace new responsibilities and play new roles. As a result, their relationship changes with politics, the citizens, their commercial rivals, and, within the organisations, between management and staff. Based on reflections about each relationship noted above, and how it has changed due to hybridity, several conclusions can be drawn.

Because of their increased hybridity, waste management services owned by local governments are now serious rivals of their commercial counterparts. This creates the dual risk of (1) public money leaking away into commercial (and thus risky) endeavours and of (2) free trade being distorted. However, at least in the cases discussed here, the first risk seems to be rather hypothetical. And, in case of the second risk, while local waste organizations that also sell their services on the marketplace might be a thorn in the side of their commercial rivals, much can be said in favour of such activities from a public interest standpoint. The first risk asks for sufficient control mechanisms to ensure the loss of public money remains a mere hypothetical risk. The second requires politicians to stick to their guns and take their role as guardians of the public interest seriously.

Hybridity also changes the relationship an organisation has with citizens: when organisations are asked to behave more business-like, they begin to see citizens as customers, who rightly demand value for money. Efficiency, effectiveness and performance become key points of interest, in itself a positive development. But there is another side to this coin, as this value-for-money approach only includes contracted services: the organisation only supplies those services it has been paid for. The cases discussed here seem to suggest that there might be a trade-off between efficiency and customer satisfaction due to hybridity.

Hybridity also dramatically alters the relationship an organisation has with its political principals, as those now have to play two new roles: that of shareholder and that of commissioning body, which generally do not come easy to politicians, and which at times will conflict. Hybridity can help to break through political inertia, but brings its own challenges. As shareholders, politicians will mostly be interested in whether an organisation can guarantee a return on investment and how high this dividend will be. Such interests can run contrary to those of a commissioning body, whose main concern is continuity of service provision. Municipalities often find playing their new roles as commissioning bodies difficult, as they lack the necessary expertise. Supervisory boards can help to provide more checks and balances, but it seems only when politics and politicians are kept out of them.

Hybridity does not leave the organisation itself untouched either, and especially alters the relationship between its management and staff. Whereas before the latter were the boss, because of hybridity and the economic and business-like values it introduces, the first takes over. This is not necessarily a bad thing, as often a lack of leadership and management can result in undesirable practices taking hold, and can give way to the development of personal fiefdoms, but it also asks for a careful approach that takes into account that cultures are hard to be managed and surely cannot change fundamentally within a short period of time.

As a general conclusion, the increased hybridity of waste management provides us with a mixed bag. There are some positive developments, but also several side effects that are less desirable. While this is often the case (there are hardly any developments in the social world which are either completely beneficial or completely catastrophic) it still tells us that we should tread with care when it comes to hybridity in waste management. After all, several important public interests are at play. This not only asks for more research on hybridity (a classic recommendation by an academic, perhaps), but surely a broad discussion about what to expect through hybridity, and how its negative side effects can be kept at bay.

References

Afval Overleg Orgaan (2002) *Borging van publieke belangen in het afvalbeheer* [*Guaranteeing public interests in waste management*], No AOO 02v-a-0006, Utrecht: AOO.

Brandsen, T. and Karré, P.M. (2011) 'Hybrid organizations: No cause for concern?', *International Journal of Public Administration*, vol 34, no 13, pp 827-36.

Brandsen, T., van de Donk, W. and Putters, K. (2005) 'Griffins or chameleons? Hybridity as a permanent and inevitable characteristic of the third sector', *International Journal of Public Administration*, vol 28, nos 9-10, pp 749-65.

Christensen, T. and Lægreid, P. (2011) *The Ashgate Research Companion to New Public Management*, Farnham: Ashgate.

Commissie Toekomstige Organisatie Afvalverwijdering (1996) *Eindrapport commissie toekomstige organisatie afvalverwijdering* [*Final report of the Commission on the Future Organisation of Waste Disposal*], Den Haag.

Dijkgraaf, E. (2004) *Regulating the Dutch waste market*, Rotterdam: Erasmus Universiteit Rotterdam.

Greve, C. (2007) *Contracting for public services*, London: Routledge.

Hall, D. (2010) *Waste management companies in Europe 2009*, London: Public Services International Research Unit.

Karré, P.M. (2011) *Heads and tails: Both sides of the coin. An analysis of hybrid organizations in the Dutch waste management sector*, The Hague: Eleven International Publishing.

Ministerie van Economische Zaken (2000) *Publieke belangen en marktordening: Liberalisering en privatisering in netwerksectoren* [*Public interests and the organisation of the market in utilities*], Den Haag: Ministerie van Economische Zaken.

Netherlands Court of Audit (2004) *Public entrepreneurship: Supervision of and reporting on public–private arrangements*, The Hague: Algemene Rekenkamer.

NL Agency (2011) *Afvalstoffenheffing 2011* [*Waste management fees 2011*], The Hague: Agentschap NL.

Pollitt, C. and Bouckaert, G. (2011) *Public management reform – A comparative analysis: New public management, governance, and the neo-Weberian state*, Oxford: Oxford University Press.

SenterNovem (2006) *De afvalmarkt 2006: Overheidsondernemingen en huishoudelijk restafval* [*State-owned enterprises and municipal waste*], Utrecht: SenterNovem.

Skelcher, C. (2007) 'Public–private partnerships and hybridity', in E. Ferlie, L.E. Lynn and C. Pollitt (eds) *The Oxford handbook of public management*, Oxford: Oxford University Press, pp 347-70.

EIGHT

Waste management companies: critical urban infrastructural services that design the sociomateriality of waste

Hervé Corvellec and Johan Hultman

Introduction

In this chapter, we demonstrate that waste management companies participate in a decisive manner in the design of the sociomateriality of waste, and that this participation gives them a particularly important role for urban development. The sociomateriality of waste refers to the way organisations and individuals engage with the materiality of waste in the course of their daily operations and everyday life (Gregson, 2009). Sociomateriality is not fixed. Instead, the sociomateriality of waste is contingent on the social understanding that people have of the nature, origins and destiny of waste as material. It encompasses different dimensions as to how waste is accepted as construction material for new houses (Bahamón and Sanjinés, 2010), how it function in art works (Vergine, 2007), or how people conceive of their responsibility towards waste (Åkesson and Ohlsson, 2006).

Waste management companies shape the sociomateriality of waste through their communicative and managerial practice. Their logistic choices determine the minutes, rhythms and paths of waste mobilities. They form a critical infrastructure that offers a service that not only brings a practical solution to the problems experienced by waste producers who wish to get rid of their waste, but waste management companies also connect the commodity and post-commodity phases of products, and bridge design, production, distribution and consumption stages to the reuse, recycling or landfill stages of materials (Leonard, 2010). In this, they make possible a functional urban life in materialist and pro-growth economies, not least by embedding their practices of waste management in societal discourses of material scarcity and global environmental responsibility.

This chapter has four main sections. First, we describe three successive Swedish post-Second World War waste governance regimes. Second, we explain how each of these regimes entails a specific sociomateriality of waste. Third, through a case study, we illustrate how waste management companies shape this sociomateriality. And fourth, we discuss the activities of waste management companies in terms of providing critical urban infrastructure services. We conclude by establishing the centrality of waste management companies for the definition of the sociomateriality of waste.

Sweden's efforts to climb the waste hierarchy

Understanding waste governance is necessary to understand the sociomateriality of waste. Sweden has developed three successive waste governance regimes (Gille, 2007) since the Second World War. In the post-war period a 'landfilling' regime to accommodate the growing production of waste dominated. The increasing amount of organic, paper and plastic waste, but also other disposables and construction material waste, was sent to landfill sites. These were traditional sites, basically holes in the ground or artificial hills. However, health-related, social, aesthetic and environmental concerns raised in the late 1960s made decision makers doubt that these landfill sites could accommodate a long-term growth in waste volume. A new waste governance regime was needed.

The rationale of the new waste governance regime, emerging in the early 1970s, was to reduce the volume of waste sent to landfill sites. To reduce volume, the responsibility of waste was entrusted to municipalities. Many launched ambitious programmes of incineration that they systematically pursued during the following decades. Essential to this was the concomitant development of municipal district heating programmes that allowed many municipally owned waste management companies to recover electricity and heat from incineration, and provided them with a steady source of income (Corvellec et al, 2012; Corvellec and Bramryd, 2012). Also essential was the rapid increase of the tax on landfill introduced in 2000, and the restrictions established in 2002 on the landfilling of combustible material, two legal measures that redirected much waste from landfills to waste-to-energy facilities. In parallel with developing waste-to-energy programmes, recycling programmes have been facilitated on a national scale. From 1994, systems for extended producers' responsibility have been introduced for a series of waste streams, starting with paper and packaging, but now also including batteries, end-of-life vehicles, and electric and electronic waste. Moreover, several municipalities have developed biological treatment capacities, an effort that the Swedish Parliament encouraged when setting the goal that nutrients should be recovered from at least a third of household biological waste by 2015.

The objective of sending less waste to landfill sites has been successful. Whereas nearly all waste was brought to landfills in 1970, it is the destiny of only 1 per cent of municipal solid waste today if one considers incineration a form of recycling, and accordingly classifies incineration ashes as recycled material. Waste-to-energy processing takes care of 49 per cent of household waste, material recovery of 36 per cent, biological treatment of 13 per cent, and the management of hazardous waste of 1 per cent (Avfall Sverige, 2011b).

A key to the success of the 'less landfilling' regime has been waste management companies' ability to transform waste into a resource. Waste-to-energy and biological treatment facilities and recycling schemes demonstrate not only that it is possible to reduce the amount of waste sent to landfill; they also show that waste has economic, environmental and social value. However, a third waste governance regime is emerging, in important respects contradictory to the idea that waste is a resource to exploit. This regime prioritises the prevention of waste. The rationale for this is that preventing the production of waste is more important in environmental terms than extracting economic value from existing waste. Central principles include a design philosophy that takes the whole product life cycle into consideration, lean modes of production to systematically reduce material spill, for example, in municipal school catering, and consumer practices that encourage thrift or that prolong the commodity phase of products, for example, repair, maintenance and second-hand retail (Avfall Sverige, 2011b). The 'waste prevention' regime is not yet as systematically developed in practice as the regime aimed at reducing landfill. In a way, it is still more a matter of ambitions, for example, Sweden's national waste plan (Naturvårdverket, 2011), than of practical solutions. But the waste prevention regime is emerging as a new societal narrative of wasting less to challenge the established societal narrative of less landfill (Corvellec and Hultman, 2012).

The emergence of this third regime is a result of Sweden's efforts to climb the European Union's (EU) waste hierarchy (European Commission, 2008a). The hierarchy ranks the desirability of five different waste management options according to their environmental impact. At the top of the hierarchy (1) are practices that aim for the prevention of waste, that is, modes of design, production and consumption that do not result in waste generation. This most preferred option is followed by (2) reuse of products, which means that products circulate in and out of the commodity phase in a way so that their function can be repeatedly fulfilled. A result of these two options is decreased material circulation. The next two steps promote the increased circulation of materials to create output with economic value: (3) recycling and composting indicates post-commodity material disassembly and sorting, after which materials can be reintroduced to industrial and biological production processes; and (4) incineration of waste with energy and heat recovery. The least desirable option (5) is landfill, which results in no significant output with economic value (Hultman and Corvellec, 2012).

The post-war 'waste governance' regime of landfilling waste corresponds to the bottom and least desirable step of the hierarchy. The 'less landfilling' regime corresponds to the steps concerned with incineration with energy and heat recovery and recycling and composting. The 'wasting less' regime corresponds to the two most desirable steps of reuse and prevention. Swedish waste management aims to reach the higher steps of the waste hierarchy (Avfall Sverige, 2011a), and such a move involves transformation of the sociomateriality of waste.

Changing the sociomateriality of waste

In a landfilling regime, the sociomateriality of waste is characterised by dissociation, separation and disappearance. The production of waste is dissociated from consumption in the sense that consumers and other waste producers do not engage with the fate of materials beyond their commodity phase. In Sweden – corresponding to the development of the welfare state and a consumption-intensive way of life – throwing things away deemed to be without value or interest was established as legitimate behaviour. The responsibility of consumers was limited to bringing waste to a collection point where waste cognitively disappeared. The rationale of waste management under such a regime is to make waste invisible and odourless, so that waste producers can physically and psychologically separate from it. Waste is considered as something inert that should be accumulated in some (remote) place.

The 'less landfilling' regime builds on waste-to-energy and recycling practices, consequently shaping a different sociomateriality of waste. This regime brings waste back to those who produced it as heat and electricity. Likewise, engaging people in nation-wide recycling practices demonstrates that waste not only has a history, but also a future. It then becomes the responsibility of each individual waste producer to ensure, through adequate and careful sorting practices, that the resource potential of waste is realised. Defined as a resource, the visibility of waste is legitimised. It also becomes increasingly embedded in local, regional and transnational economies. Waste management companies regularly inform their customers of how much paper, metal and plastic they have recycled, and how many new newspapers, cars or plastic bottles this corresponds to. For example, all schoolchildren in the city of Helsingborg are introduced to the basics of waste management and taken on a tour of the municipal waste management facility and old landfill site. Correspondingly, the city of Malmö takes pride on its website for tourists in how it addresses waste by making an issue out of the fact that one of its recent residential projects has vacuum waste chutes to minimise heavy traffic (Malmö Tourism, 2011). The city also underscores the initiative to collect all food waste in Malmö for use in the production of biogas for city buses (Malmö Tourism, 2011). Under the 'less landfilling' regime, waste is subjected to the logic of material effectiveness: it is a resource that should be systematically exploited instead of being uselessly wasted.

The 'wasting less' regime rests on yet a different sociomateriality of waste: waste is something that should not become, which makes waste a problematic materiality. The management of waste is not to make waste disappear, as in the landfilling regime. Nor is it to optimise the use of waste, as in the 'less landfilling' regime. Instead, waste management is the systematic effort to prevent the existence of waste. Waste is a sign of inefficiency. It is a failure to be avoided and, as all failures, a possible motive of blame (Hawkins, 2006).

Increasing quantities of waste, growing concerns for the environmental impact of landfill sites and incineration, intensifying political demands for the recycling of waste and fears of future material shortages have resulted in a series of changes in the social and material presence of waste in capitalist consumer economies. Waste is no longer a disturbing by-product of consumption that waste producers pay to have removed. It has become an object of both desire and avoidance, open for political determination and everyday attention. It has become a source of legal and moral responsibility. There is a growing recognition that the concept of waste is, in important ways, becoming nonsensical: 'there is no waste' claims the trade organisation Swedish Waste Management (Avfall Sverige, 2011a).

Waste management organisations have played a decisive role in these successive redefinitions of the sociomateriality of waste, from a regime of invisibility to one of failure via one of resource. Contemporary waste management organisations are diversified organisations that operate a wide range of collection and recycling technologies. They systematically market the products of their processes, for example, energy or materials, and they counsel their customers on how to reduce their production of waste and optimise the management of waste that is nevertheless produced. They work to secure their local symbolic and legislative legitimacy in an increasingly deregulated and internationalised industry, and systematically embed their management of waste in the emerging discourse of sustainable production and consumption. They weave the mobilities and transformations of waste tightly into the social and urban fabric, thereby connecting waste to contemporary politics of consumption.

The European waste hierarchy requires waste companies to find innovative ways to prevent, disassemble and reassemble the materiality of waste (Hultman and Corvellec, 2012). This leads these companies to develop their activities vertically, for example, by articulating their services with corporate cradle-to-cradle design and production strategies (McDonough and Braungart, 2009). They also need to develop their activities horizontally and coordinate actions across institutional and organisational boundaries (European Commission, 1999, 2008b; Watson et al, 2008). The value-creating potential of waste companies rests on their ability to power material circulation.

Designing sociomateriality in practice

The case of a Swedish municipality-owned waste company illustrates how waste management companies influence how waste producers define the materiality of waste, how this definition is embedded in larger cultural representations and how it is inscribed in urbanity. NSR (Nordvästra Skånes Renhållnings AB [Northwest Scania Recycling Ltd]) is a waste management company co-owned by six municipalities in the region of Northwest Skåne in southern Sweden. Its owners have endowed NSR with a legal responsibility for the collection and treatment of waste in the region. This legal responsibility gives the company a monopoly on household waste within the jurisdiction of its owners, with the exception of the waste streams that belong to the systems of extended producers' responsibility. NSR also has the possibility of bidding for the collection and treatment of industrial waste up to a certain percentage of its turnover, but then in competition with other private or publicly owned waste management companies (Corvellec et al, 2012; Corvellec and Bramryd, 2012).

NSR is characterised by its focus on recycling and the biological treatment of waste. This commitment to recycling and biogas production has led NSR to repeatedly inform the public about the benefits for households to sort their waste. The company stresses that sorting waste correctly makes it possible for much waste to be recycled, with the subtext that this separation has to be performed exactly as NSR instructs. To realise this demand, NSR has developed a system of multifractions neighbourhood collection for household waste. NSR has designed bins that are specially designed for this system, and NSR's rhythm of waste collection. NSR teaches waste producers how to look at their waste, how to recognise what belongs to each fraction (for example, paper as opposed to cardboard, or hard plastic as opposed to soft plastic), how to use brown paper bags to collect food waste, when to take out the bins and other technicalities (NSR, 2012a). This system offers waste producers a service that fits their (experienced) time limitations, in particular by reducing their need for transportation. At the same time it gives them the possibility of negotiating their environmental consciousness with only minimal efforts, leaving consumption practices out of the equation. Along with using public transportation, recycling waste is among the contributions that urban dwellers think of first when trying to make their way of living more sustainable (see, for example, Beavan, 2009).

To run its waste management service with efficiency and thus reach its objectives, NSR is dependent on the collaboration of waste producers. Waste management imposes collective choices on individual practices. If waste producers are to engage in recycling practices, they need to experience systems of recycling practices (Gregson, 2009) as reliable and meaningful. Backed by its legal monopoly of household waste within the legislation of its owners, NSR has leverage to shape the behaviour of households. It is systematically working on getting people to subject themselves fully to the discursive and practical order of governmentality (Foucault, 1991; Dean, 1999; Skålen et al, 2006) that the company has designed, with clear sets of categories, classification, priorities, moral obligations, rewards and penalties.

NSR keeps reminding waste producers that food waste is nothing to throw away with unsorted waste, but something valuable to separate for biogas production. Food waste is designated, framed, priced and embedded in societal narrative as well as everyday practices. NSR transforms wasted food items from ambiguously, undefined things into named, understood, transparent and performative materialities (Knappett, 2008). NSR gives a social life to waste things (Appadurai, 1986), and turns a thing of repulsion into an object of desire.

The message about the future social life of food waste as fuel for mobility is passed along in brochures, through advertisement campaigns on buses and street furniture, and in messages posted on the company's website. People are told that biogas is 'an environment friendly and renewable fuel' that is 'at the centre of the cycle' (NSR, ca 2008c), 'City buses in Helsingborg run on NSR biogas' and '[d]omestic foodwaste upgraded to vehicle fuel are the best waste dump in the world' (NSR, ca 2008a). Separating food waste is represented as a way to assume environmental responsibility by bettering urban life and mitigating climate change. NSR underscores that since it produces bio-fertilisers distributed to local farmers, separating food waste is also a way to give back to the nearby fields the nutrients that these fields have offered and now need back (NSR, ca 2008b). The challenge for NSR is to convince the public that it is legitimate to demand from every household that it enters and accepts being locked into the practical order of waste handling that the company has designed.

The same is true of NSR's relationships with companies, except that companies are not included in NSR's monopoly on household waste, and can choose among public and private waste management companies. They have to be persuaded. To attract larger companies or companies with environmental ambitions, NSR has designed 'a comprehensive waste management contract, with a personal contact, closeness to services and an overview of waste management situation' (authors' translation; NSR, 2011a). The service consists of an in-depth analysis of the customer's internal waste producing processes, custom waste prevention separation and collection solutions, and information material. Smaller companies are offered 'an effective management of waste streams with custom waste collection and proximity to efficient service' (authors' translation; NSR, 2011b). Moreover, NSR offers to act as a consultant to businesses throughout the region for hazardous waste, 'offering the services of its chemists and safety advisers in the classification and handling of all categories of hazardous waste, with the exception of radioactive waste' (NSR, 2007: 11).

NSR's purpose with companies is the same as with households: to encourage interest for waste, provide practical guidance about how to understand waste, inscribe waste in the waste producer's economic and environmental concerns, bring practical solutions to these concerns, suggest appropriate behaviour to the waste producer, including rhythms and places of collection, set up systems of rewards and penalties, and create social, economic and environmental satisfaction. Thereby, NSR tames the force of things (Bennett, 2004) to endow waste with economic and environmental value. The company designs a sociomateriality of waste that answers to its mission – as a regional economic and environmental infrastructure – to offer the regional business community competitive environmental and waste management systems (Helsingborg Stad – Kommunfullmäktige, 2005). In its 2008 annual report (NSR, 2009), NSR claims to answer to this mission in the following terms:

> NSR shall be a company that, in collaboration with private actors and the municipalities in Northwest Scania, manages household and industrial waste in a way that is cost efficient and service-minded, but also environmentally efficient and conceived in accordance with the current legislation as well as actual research and development in the field of waste management. The company shall also contribute to the development of new waste management and recycling methods, promote regional growth and development, and create environmental improvements, for example through collaborations with universities and regional businesses.

NSR embeds services in future-oriented narratives of regional competitiveness and of regional development toward sustainability. In its annual report (NSR, 2012b), NSR is also careful to inscribe its activities in a narrative of European efforts at minimising waste. Waste management has the capacity to bridge micro- and macro-societal levels and to aggregate individual choices into collective achievements or misdeeds. These regional and global narratives prolong and develop the micro-narratives about the moral economy of duty, responsibility and reward that describe the practicalities of a correct waste management for waste producers. Through these narratives, NSR promises citizens in the Helsingborg region that they can actually co-create the development of more sustainable and liveable cities and regions. The sociomateriality of waste shaped by a critical infrastructural service connects spatial categories, organisational levels and everyday life.

Waste management as a critical urban infrastructure service

From having been end-of-line sites for the treatment of waste in the landfilling regime, waste management companies are increasingly involved in developing schemes of material circulation that interfere with the dominant politics of production and consumption. Because they design, offer, deliver, price, narrate and develop waste management services to waste producers, waste management organisations are an infrastructure providing a critical service for urban life.

Waste management is an infrastructure in that it is part of the 'the basic, underlying structure or character' of a society (Calhoun, 2002). It is an activity that is more important to the economy than its mere turnover and how many people it employs, and more important to social life than its share of political programmes. Like other infrastructures, waste management is an 'essential background for other economic activities in modern economies' (Black et al, 2009: 229). It is something that is 'needed to support commerce as well as economic and residential development' (Black and Garner, 1999: 784) and that is 'promoting optimum opportunities for competition and living standards for society and its members' (Evert, 2011: 324).

More specifically, waste management can be considered a critical infrastructure. The notion of critical infrastructures refers to 'systems that provide critical support services to a country, geographic area for a corporate entity; when they fail, there is potentially a large cost in human life, the environment or economic markets' (Egan, 2007: 4). In other words, critical infrastructures are 'systems, facilities, and assets so vital that, if destroyed or incapacitated, would disrupt the security, economy, health, safety, or welfare of the public' (American Society of Civil Engineers's Critical Infrastructure Guidance Task Committee, 2009: 56). And even though public authorities do not usually list waste management among critical infrastructures (Commission of the European Communities, 2004), one can easily acknowledge that waste management operations belong to the 'physical and information technology facilities, networks, services and assets that, if disrupted or destroyed, would have a serious impact on the health, safety, security or economic well-being of citizens or the effective functioning of governments in EU countries' (p 3), which is the European Programme for Critical Infrastructure Protection's definition of critical infrastructures (European Commission, 2006).

Consumption-intensive societies cannot function without waste management systems, just as they cannot exist without roads, railroads and airports, a water supply and sewers, electricity production and grids, and telecommunications, but also institutional, social or recreational infrastructures. The spectacle of the collapse of waste management in Naples (Nicola, 2009), scavengers of open landfill sites in 'third world' countries (L. Walker et al, 2010), or, in a slightly different register, the first final repository for nuclear waste (Madsen, 2010), all bear witness to the criticality of waste management: it is an activity that cannot fail.

As infrastructure, waste management therefore delivers a critical service to households, businesses and, more generally, urbanity. In Sweden, households and businesses can safely *assume* that waste collection and treatment will take care of the waste they produce in the course of their activities. Waste management companies promise, regardless of bad weather or other impediments, to assume responsibility for the production of waste. They have strategically combined a broad range of distributed resources and competences, such as technological and marketing expertise, and unique environmental permits delivered by national environmental authorities.

Waste management is thus a service in the lexical sense of doing something 'for the benefit or at the command of another' and 'in an effort for human welfare or betterment' (Webster and Gove, 1971: 2075). People wish to get rid of their waste, and waste management companies help them to do so. Waste management companies also offer a service to households and industries in the more theoretical sense of service marketing literature. Waste management is a service in the sense of being a process consisting of a series of activities where a number of different types of resources are used in direct interaction with a customer, so that a solution is found to a customer's problem (Grönroos, 2000). Likewise, waste management is a service in the sense of being the application of specialised competences (knowledge and skills), through deeds, processes and performances by one entity for the benefit of another entity or the entity itself (Lusch and Vargo, 2006).

This service to waste producers is also a service that secures urban life. It is not only an urban service in the sense given to the expression by Baer (1985: 886) of 'one which serves the public interest by accomplishing one or more of the following purposes: preserving life, liberty and property; and promoting public enlightenment, happiness and domestic tranquillity and the general welfare'. An urban service is not merely a service to the urban public; it is a service to the city per se because it exists for the benefit of the urban condition. To paraphrase service marketing literature (Lusch and Vargo, 2006), an urban service is the application of specialised competences (knowledge and skills), through deeds, processes and performances by one entity or several entities for the benefit of urbanity.

The social and political organisation of cities rests on the organisation of the various flows that constitute urbanity, for example, transportation, water supply and sewage, or information (Latham, 2009). Waste is one of these flows, and organising the mobility of waste is a condition of urban life. This mobility is not limited by city boundaries. The relegation of waste to non-urban landfill illustrates the domination that cities exert on non-urban territories where the demand for food, water and other essentials is doubled by external demands for the storage of urban overflow.

The intertwining of urban and non-urban areas through material economies is a direct expression of the promise for a better society that characterises modernity (Kaika, 2005). Waste management is part of this promise. When the international waste management company REMONDIS (2012) puts banners on its website that state 'No crude oil – No modern convenience' or 'No copper – No cars', it not only promotes its recycling activities; it also promises that waste management operates to serve modern urban society. The EU does the same when it promotes its waste hierarchy (European Commission, 2008) as a governance tool for waste management policies: a careful scheme of prevention, reuse, recycling, incineration with energy recovery and landfills is to ensure the sustainability of consumption-intensive urban modes of living. Waste management is at the service of cities and is of critical importance for urbanity.

Conclusion

The organisational practices (Chia and MacKay, 2007; Gherardi, 2009; Corradi et al, 2010) of Swedish waste management companies establish a sociomaterial order of waste that materialise an idea (Strandvad, 2011) of sustainability. They link the micro-practices of households and businesses to the destiny of the region, its cities and the nation (Swedish Environmental Protection Agency, 2005). This sociomaterial order precedes the circulation of waste between people, waste-producing companies and waste management companies in the sense that it is a condition for this circulation to run smoothly. At the same time, this sociomaterial order derives from the everyday practices of waste: carrying the brown paper bag for food waste to the correct bin, collection trucks regularly criss-crossing the cities and the countryside, waste reduction strategies that corporations put into place, and campaigns where waste management companies represent recycling as civic mindedness. One of the main strategic challenges for waste management companies is to imprint on the subjectivity of their public, as they imagine it (L. Walker et al, 2010), a rich and diversified sociomateriality of waste that fits the plans of their owners and their own corporate plans.

Waste management companies help design the sociomateriality of waste through their planning, communicative, pricing, logistic, marketing, recycling and consulting practices. They have the potential to shape a material economy that addresses all of the five steps of the European waste hierarchy, although with significant differences between companies. They articulate representations of sustainable ways to handle waste; they point at individual and collective responsibilities; they give new names and new identities to what traditionally is called waste or rubbish; they devise new rhythms and routes for waste mobilities, including sales of recycled materials and reuse solutions; and they provide waste prevention advice to decouple waste production from economic growth. Waste management companies connect the production of waste to the politics of production and consumption in consumer societies.

How waste management companies devise and combine practices of landfilling, incineration, energy recovery, recycling, reuse and waste prevention is central to the politics of consumption and sustainable urban development. These companies are not alone in designing the sociomateriality of waste. Their impact on this sociomateriality is mitigated by a long range of symbolic, legal, political and institutional influences. For example, their definition of what waste is and how it should be processed is directly affected by claims of environmental injustice, prompted by the spectacle of the illegal export of hazardous waste to 'third world' countries. But waste management companies are pivotal in the definition of the sociomateriality of waste in that they are the ones that *in practice* order waste. Considering the environmental significance of waste, this is why waste management companies are critical to a sustainable urban future.

Acknowledgements

This study is part of the research project, 'Organising critical infrastructure services – A case study of waste research' (www.ism.lu.se/oki) under the Winning Services Research Programme financed by Vinnova, the Swedish Governmental Agency for Innovation Systems. We are most grateful to our respondents at NSR for the careful attention that they have shown us.

References

Åkesson, L. and Ohlsson, V. (2006) *Överflöd: Mellan minnesvärt och bortglömt* [*Overflows: Between memorable and forgotten*], Lund: Kulturen i Lund.

American Society of Civil Engineers's Critical Infrastructure Guidance Task Committee (2009) 'Guiding principles for critical infrastructure', *Civil Engineering*, vol 79, pp 56-61.

Appadurai, A. (1986) 'Commodities and the politics of value', in A. Appadurai (ed) *The social life of things: Commodities in cultural perspective*, Cambridge: Cambridge University Press, pp 34-43.

Avfall Sverige (2011a) *Det finns inget avfall: En vision för Avfall Sverige* [*There is no waste: A vision for Swedish waste management*], Malmö: Avfall Sverige.

Avfall Sverige (2011b) *Svensk Avfallshantering 2011* [*Waste management in Sweden*], Malmö: Avfall Sverige.

Baer, W.C. (1985) 'Just what is an urban service, anyway?', *Journal of Politics*, vol 47, pp 881-98.

Bahamón, A. and Sanjinés, M.C. (2010) *Rematerial: From waste to architecture*, New York: W.W. Norton & Co.

Beavan, C. (2009) *No impact man*, New York: Picador.

Bennett, J. (2004) 'The force of things: Steps toward an ecology of matter', *Political Theory*, vol 32, pp 347-72.

Black, H.C. and Garner, B. (1999) *Black's law dictionary*, St Paul, MN: Thomson West.

Black, J., Hashimzade, N. and Myles, G.D. (2009) *A dictionary of economics*, Oxford: Oxford University Press.

Calhoun, C.J. (2002) *Dictionary of the social sciences*, New York: Oxford University Press.

Chia, R. and MacKay, B. (2007) 'Post-processual challenges for the emerging strategy-as-practice perspective: Discovering strategy in the logic of practice', *Human Relations*, vol 60, pp 217-42.

Commission of the European Communities (COM(2004) 702 final) *Communication from the Commission to the Council and the European Parliament – Critical infrastructure protection in the fight against terrorism*, Brussels: Commission of the European Communities.

Commission of the European Communities (2005) *Green Paper on a European programme for critical infrastructure protection*, Brussels: Commission of the European Communities.

Corradi, G., Gherardi, S. and Verzelloni, L. (2010) 'Through the practice lens: Where is the bandwagon of practice-based studies heading?', *Management Learning*, vol 41, pp 265-83.

Corvellec, H. and Bramryd T. (2012). 'The multiple market-exposure of waste management companies: A case study of two Swedish municipally owned companies', *Waste Management*, vol 32, no 9, pp 1722-7.

Corvellec, H. and Hultman, J. (2012) 'From "less landfilling" to "wasting less" – societal narratives, socio-materiality and organizations', *Journal of Organizational Change Management*, vol 25, pp 297-314.

Corvellec, H., Bramryd, T. and Hultman, J. (2012) 'The business model of solid waste management in Sweden – a case study of two municipally-owned companies', *Waste Management & Research*, vol 30, no 5, pp 512-18.

Dean, M. (1999) *Governmentality: Power and rule in modern society*, Thousand Oaks, CA: Sage Publications.

Egan, M.J. (2007) 'Anticipating future vulnerability: Defining characteristics of increasingly critical infrastructure-like systems', *Journal of Contingencies and Crisis Management*, vol 15, pp 4-17.

European Commission (1999) *EU focus on waste management*, Luxembourg: Office for Official Publications of the European Communities.

European Commission (2008a) '2008/98/EC. Directive 2008/98/EC of the European Parliament and the Council on waste and repealing certain documents', *Official Journal of the European Union L 312/3*, Brussels: European Commission.

European Commission (2008b) *EU waste policy. The story behind the strategy*, Brussels: European Commission (http://ec.europa.eu/environment/waste/strategy.htm).

Evert, K.-J. (ed) (2011) *Encyclopedic dictionary of landscape and urban planning: Multilingual reference book in English, Spanish, French, and German*, Stuttgart: Springer & International Federation of Landscape Architects – Federation Internationale des Architectes Paysagistes.

Foucault, M. (1991) 'Governmentality', in G. Burchell, C. Gordon and P. Miller (eds) *The Foucault effect: Studies in governmentality*, Chicago, IL: University of Chicago Press, pp 87-104.

Gherardi, S. (2009) 'Practice? It's a matter of taste!', *Management Learning*, vol 40, pp 535-50.

Gille, Z. (2007) *From the cult of waste to the trash heap of history*, Bloomington, IN: Indiana University Press.

Gregson, N. (2009) 'Challenging assumptions: Recycling as policy and assemblage', *Geography*, vol 94, pp 61-5.

Grönroos, C. (2000) *Service management and marketing: A customer relationship management approach*, Chichester: Wiley.

Hawkins, G. (2006) *The ethics of waste: How we relate to rubbish*, Lanham, MD: Rowman & Littlefield.

Helsingborg Stad – Kommunfullmäktige (2005) *Ägardirektiv för NSR (Nordvästra Skånes Renhållnings AB)* [*Owners' directive*], Helsingborg: Helsingborg Stad.

Hultman, J. and Corvellec, H. (2012) 'The European waste hierarchy: from the socio-materiality of waste to a politics of consumption', *Environment & Planning A*, vol 44, no 10, pp 2413-27.

Kaika, M. (2005) *City of flows: Modernity, nature, and the city*, New York: Routledge.

Knappett, C. (2008) 'The neglected networks of material agency: artefacts, pictures and texts', in C. Knappett and L. Malafouris (eds) *Material agency: Towards a non-anthropocentric approach*, New York: Springer, pp 139-56.

Latham, A. (2009) *Key concepts in urban geography*, Los Angeles, CA: Sage Publications.

Leonard, A. (2010) *The story of stuff: How our problem with overconsumption is trashing the planet, our communities and our health – and what to do about it*, London: Constable.

Lusch, R.F. and Vargo, S.L. (2006) *The service-dominant logic of marketing: Dialog, debate, and directions*, Armonk, NY: M.E. Sharpe.

McDonough, W. and Braungart, M. (2009) *Cradle to cradle: Remaking the way we make things*, London: Vintage.

Madsen, M. (director) (2010) *Into eternity* [Documentary], Copenhagen: Magic Hours Films.

Malmö Tourism (2011) *Making sustainability reality in Malmö*, Malmö (www.malmotown.com/en/press/articles/making-sustainability-reality-in-malmo).

Naturvårdverket (Swedish Environmental Protection Agency) (2011) *Remissutgåva 2011-09-12 – Från avfallshantering till resurshushållning: Sveriges avfallsplan 2012-2017* [*Preliminary version 2011-09-12 – From waste management to resource management: Sweden's national waste plan 2012-2017*], Stockholm: Naturvårdsverket.

Nicola, A. (director) (2009) *Una montagna di balle* [*Wasting Naples; documentary*], Naples: Insu TV.

NSR (Nordvästra Skånes Renhållnings AB) (2007) *Putting the environment first*, Helsingborg: Nordvästra Skånes Renhållnings AB.

NSR (2009) *Årsredovisning 2008* [*Annual report 2008*], Helsingborg: NSR.

NSR (2011a) *Helkund hos NSR* [*Total customer at NSR*], Helsingborg: NSR (www.nsr.se/Default.aspx?ID=4699).

NSR (2011b) *NSR® Xakt*, Helsingborg: NSR (www.nsr.se/Default.aspx?ID=4704).

NSR (2012a) *Det är lätt att sortera rätt!* [*It is easy to sort waste!*], Helsingborg: NSR (www.bastad.se/Documents/).

NSR (2012b) *NSR för 'Europa minskar avfallet'* [*NSR is for 'Europe reduces its waste'*], Helsingborg: NSR.

NSR (2008a) 'Domestic foodwaste upgraded to vehicle fuel are the best waste dump in the world' [Leaflet], Helsingborg: NSR.

NSR (2008b) 'NSR biogödsel' ['NSR bio-fertliser'] [Leaflet], Helsingborg: NSR.

NSR (2008c) *Biogas: The fuel at the center of the cycle*, Helsingborg: NSR.

REMONDIS (2012) *Water, raw materials and energy – for now and for the future*, Lünen: REMONDIS AG & Co KG (www.remondis.com/index.php?id=304&L=1).

Skålen, P., Fellesson, M. and Fougere, M. (2006) 'The governmentality of marketing discourse', *Scandinavian Journal of Management*, vol 22, pp 275-91.

Strandvad, S.M. (2011) 'Materializing ideas: A socio-material perspective on the organizing of cultural production', *European Journal of Cultural Studies*, vol 14, pp 283-97.

Swedish Environmental Protection Agency (2005) *A strategy for sustainable waste management: Sweden's waste plan*, Stockholm: Naturvårdsverket.

Walker, L., Harley, K. and Jardim, J. (directors) (2010) *Waste land* [Documentary], London and Rio de Janeiro: Almega Projects and O2 Filmes.

Watson, M., Bulkeley, H. and Hudson, R. (2008) 'Unpicking environmental policy integration with tales from waste management', *Environment and Planning C, Government and Policy*, vol 26, pp 481-98.

Webster, N. and Gove, P.B. (1971) *Webster's third new international dictionary of the English language*, Springfield, MA: Merriam.

Vergine, L. (2007) *When trash becomes art: Trash, rubbish, mongo*, Milan: Skira.

Part IV

Waste and environmental, economic and social justice

NINE

Cairo's contested waste: the Zabaleen's local practices and privatisation policies

Wael Fahmi and Keith Sutton

Introduction

This chapter takes up several themes and issues closely relevant to this book's central focus on organising waste in cities. A major theme concerns the conflict between Cairo's rubbish collectors' low-technology approach to solid waste management and disposal by the Zabaleen, and a high-technology approach carried out by large companies employing wage labour. This theme is related to Leonard's study of the Irish community narratives of mobilisation and struggle against state regional waste plans (see Chapter Ten), as the Zabaleen's case study raises such questions as, can a grassroots indigenous system of recycling waste resist being taken over by a supposedly modern large-scale privatised system? What are the possibilities of local–global partnership? Related conflictual issues involve a marginal society versus a mainstream economic efficiency situation, the Zabaleen society with its embedded rural values versus urban large-scale profit-maximising businesses, and poorer lower-class Zabaleen waste collectors versus middle-class demands for regular efficient waste collection and street cleaning. Another theme that is touched on involves the conflicts, actual and potential, between centralising government ministries and various non-governmental organisations (NGOs), local and international, seeking to foster improvements in the Zabaleen economy and society. Given the recent contribution of such NGOs, can they play a positive role in this new situation of privatisation and big company involvement? What is the contribution of local NGOs such as the Association for the Protection of the Environment (APE) and Environmental Quality International (EQI) as community advocates and of the *wahiya* as contractors to the Zabaleen's cause over the relocation of recycling activities to Eastern Cairo's new settlements? This issue relates to the role of NGOs in the governance of waste and the different modes of organising waste referred to earlier in Karré's study of the Dutch hybridisation of waste management (see Chapter Seven).

This chapter provides a historical review of the Zabaleen community, taking into account the early 1980s World Bank-funded Zabaleen Environmental Development Programme (ZEDP), coordinated by local NGO EQI (Fahmi, 2005). After introducing the Zabaleen rubbish recycling system, the next section discusses current plans to change drastically the solid waste management system for Cairo and the consequences of relocating the Zabaleen's settlement and recycling activities. Nevertheless the chapter examines these issues, employing local narratives recorded during focus group interviews and reactions to the threat of forced eviction as a result of potential state-controlled gentrification programmes for urban development and land speculation in the area.

Ethnographic techniques of open-ended interviews were administered, in 2004 and 2009, with 40 primary stakeholder local rubbish collectors (with heads of households) and five community leaders (representatives of the Garbage Collectors Association, Gammiya) in the Muqattam settlement. Qualitative data and narratives were gathered during focus group discussions dealing with their attitudes towards the privatisation programme and relocation plans in relation to the future of their recycling enterprises, community livelihood and social cohesion and pig-rearing activities, particularly since the 2009 swine flu pandemic and the slaughtering of their pigs. Informal discussions were carried out with five secondary stakeholder agencies: Cairo Cleaning and Beautification Authority (CCBA), Egyptian Environmental Affairs Agency (EEAA); multinational waste management companies, and with local NGOs; Community and Institutional Development (CID); and the Association for the Protection of the Environment (APE). Secondary stakeholders' narratives expressed issues related to the privatisation project's political achievement and its contribution to technical improvement within the 'Garbage City', and community empowerment and networking and environmental awareness among the Zabaleen.

The study findings highlighted the adverse effects of the privatisation of waste management systems on the sustainability of the Zabaleen's associated recycling economy. The consumption of Cairo's sites of waste collection and sorting has opened new sociopolitical spaces for conflict between multinational companies and the Zabaleen's traditional system. This is further indicated in the way Cairo's waste materials have been subjected to new claims and conflicts, as they are seen as a 'commodity' by global capital entrepreneurs and multinational corporations, and as a source of 'livelihood' by the disadvantaged and marginalised Zabaleen population.

Various authors have noted the central, but often unacknowledged, role of informal waste collectors within municipal solid waste management systems. Accordingly, in order to achieve sustainability within waste management systems, the state should formally recognise the significant role played by waste collectors and other informal actors. Visser and Theron (2009) have argued for the need to promote alternatives to private sector models while improving the conditions of those currently working in the informal waste management sector. Nzeadibe (2009) indicated that the state's failure to acknowledge and engage with the informal waste collectors meant that interventions to transform the waste management system have unintended consequences and ultimately cannot succeed.

Closely relevant to the Zabaleen's case study is the Vincentian Missionaries' (1998) development of a federation of scavengers (waste collectors/pickers) who live close to a major solid waste dump (Payatas) in Quezon City, the Philippines. The Foundation and other NGOs have supported scavengers and later facilitated a study tour to the Zabaleen waste management system in Cairo to allow consideration of a possible technology transfer. Relating the Payatas' experience to the Zabaleen system paved the way for the formulation of a Payatas Environmental Development Programme, which advocated an alternative waste management system to open dumping, and involved setting up a community-based materials recovery centre, harnessing the waste-picking and recycling skills of scavengers and micro-entrepreneurs, and further supplementing these skills with environmentally friendly technology for solid waste processing and composting. The materials recovery centre was not conceived as an industrial entity but as organised clusters of community-based enterprises involved in solid waste recycling or product-enhancing activities. A successful savings and credit programme was initiated to fund micro-enterprises and social needs, including a housing programme. The Federation has also increased the scavengers' capacity to negotiate with local authorities and other government agencies.

History of the Zabaleen rubbish collectors

About 100 years ago, a group of migrants from the Dakhla oasis in Egypt's western desert region settled in downtown Cairo. This group, known as the *wahiya* (singular, *wahi*), or people of the oasis, assumed sole responsibility for the collection and disposal of Cairo's household waste. Initially working under contract, the *wahiya* paid the buildings' owners an initial sum, and then collected monthly fees from the tenants. They later collaborated with another group of migrants, the rubbish collectors (*Zabaleen*), who came to Cairo in the 1930s and 1940s, from El Badary district in Assiut in southern Egypt. They purchased the waste for use as fodder for their pig farming. Since then, the Zabaleen community has emerged as rubbish collectors-recyclers, settling in makeshift settlements at the western and northern fringes of Cairo metropolitan region. They have maintained ties with their rural origins, preserving their community organisation by intermarrying and living in extended family situations. There was therefore a distinction between the *wahiya* and the rubbish collectors (singular, *zabal*; also called *zarraba*, singular, *zarrab*). The latter collected rubbish on donkey-pulled carts and pickup trucks accompanied by their children or siblings (see Figure 9.1). Female and younger members of the family divided the rubbish into up to 16 different types, sorting out recyclables, including making use of organic waste for feeding their pigs. Obtaining organic waste for pig rearing was perhaps more important for the Zabaleen than initially thought, since pig meat was sold to big tourist facilities. In addition, the Zabaleen sold sorted secondary materials such as paper, tin, rags, glass and plastic materials to middlemen. The *wahiya* who retained control over the access and collection rights to the rubbish, act as middlemen between the Zabaleen and Cairo's households. The Zabaleen, typically, had no share in the monthly fees paid by those residents, while being obliged to pay the *wahiya* in order to gain access to the waste.

In 1989 an agreement between the *wahiya* and the Zabaleen resulted in the establishment of new mechanised companies for waste collection. Groups of Zabaleen were contracted by the *wahiya* to collect and dispose of municipal solid waste. By the early 1990s the authorities introduced a new mechanisation system to transport solid waste, and with no governmental financial assistance being provided, the Zabaleen had to acquire capital to purchase trucks through personal cash savings, selling remaining small plots of land or houses in their ancestral village, or getting credit loans. Although the municipal sanitation service and the Zabaleen have long shared responsibility for waste collection, the formation of the EPC established the *wahiya* and the Zabaleen as key participants in the local government's programme to upgrade waste management in Cairo. The *wahiya* administer the system, market the company's services, collect household charges and supervise service deliveries (Assaad and Garas, 1994). Figure 9.2 shows the storage of bags of sorted materials ready for recycling as well as the increasingly upgraded buildings used for both residences and recycling businesses.

Figure 9.1: Rubbish collector (Zabal)

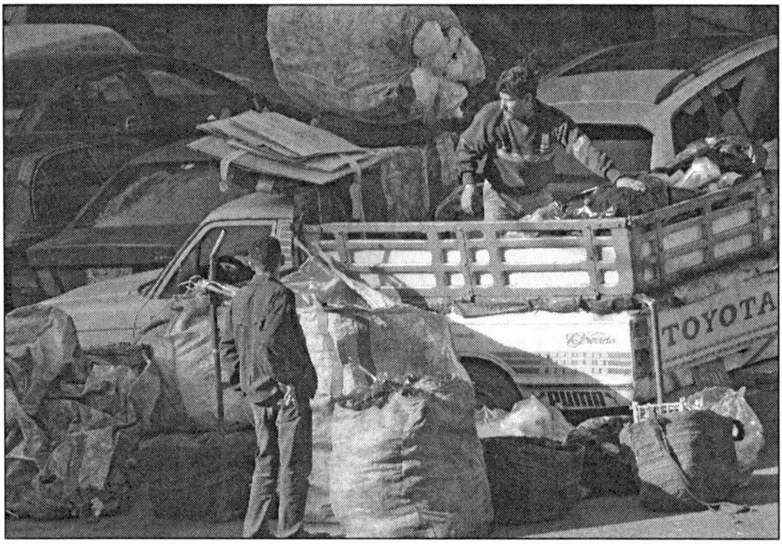

Figure 9.3 illustrates the location of the Zabaleen's main settlement between the Muqattam mountain and the long-established informal settlement of Manshiet Nasser. It also demonstrates the relative proximity of the 'Garbage City' to Cairo's business and administrative centres and to its historic cultural core in Islamic Cairo.

It is estimated that the Zabaleen informally handled one third of Cairo's waste from 14 million people, mainly from the poorer districts (Golia, 2004). The Zabaleen collected up to 3,000 tonnes of waste every day, with 85 per cent being recycled directly through micro-enterprises that generate jobs and incomes for the local community. According to a local NGO, Community and Institutional Development (CID), the average monthly wage for the waste-handling worker in Muqattam ranged from LE 360 to LE 450 (US$1 = LE 6 Egyptian pounds, January 2012 rates). The highest paid workers were those in the recycling industries, while the lowest paid were in the collection and transportation of waste. Within the Zabaleen Muqattam settlement, nearly 700 families owned collection enterprises, 200 owned and operated small and medium-scale recycling enterprises, and 120 owned trading enterprises, in addition to maintenance workshops and community-based service businesses (Assaad and Garas, 1994; Motaal, 1996). These micro-entrepreneurs have invested an estimated LE 2.1 million in purchasing trucks, plastic granulators, paper compactors, cloth grinders, aluminium smelters and tin processors. The Zabaleen

Figure 9.2: Zabaleen, 'Garbage City'

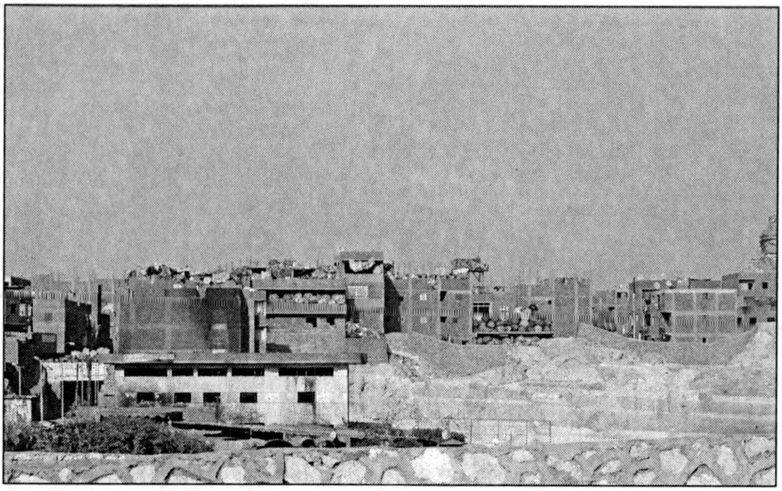

Figure 9.3: Location of the Muqattam Zabaleen settlement

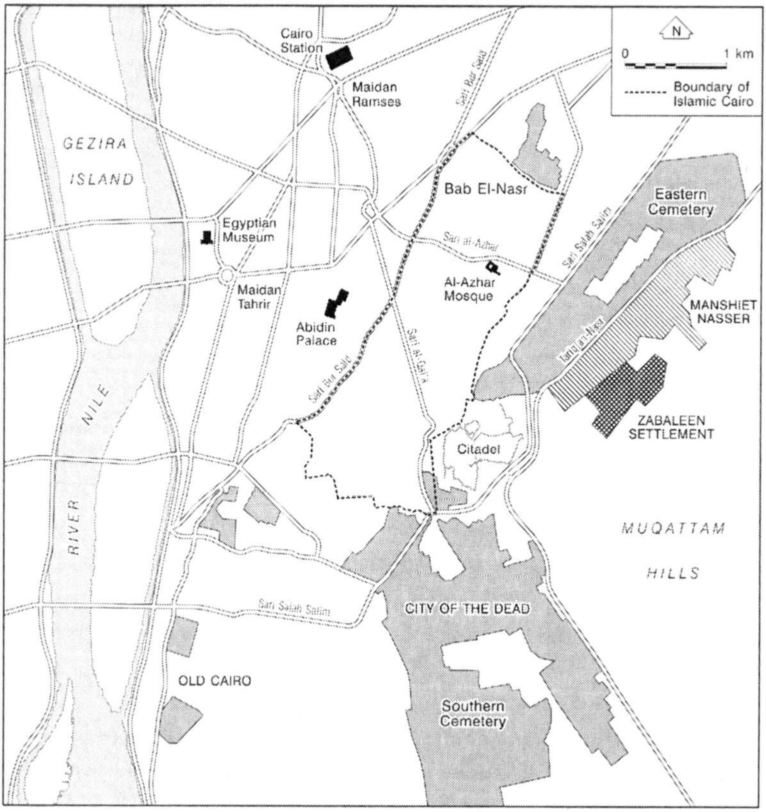

have greatly improved the capacity of Cairo to manage its solid waste, at minimal cost to the city administration, as their recycling methods for handling plastic, paper, cardboard, glass, metal and fabrics were constantly being upgraded and diversified.

Privatisation of Cairo's waste management system

In June 2002, the Zabaleen began losing their licenses as international waste management companies started taking over Cairo's waste collection routes (see Figure 9.4). While the Spanish companies FCC, Urbaser and Enser signed 15-year contracts worth US$25 million a year to manage waste in the eastern and western zones of Cairo, AMA of Italy and the Egyptian Arab Contractors won a joint 15-year contract, worth US$11.5 million a year, to operate within northern Cairo. Spanish and Italian companies, FCC and Jacorossi, signed a US$7.6 million 15-year contract to manage waste collection in the Dokki, Agouza and Imbaba districts of Giza. The contract required that International Environment Services (IES), a subsidiary of Jacorossi, would handle waste collection on a door-to-door basis, replicating the Zabaleen's system. Despite such initial success, Giza has faced problems in its transition to a privatised management system, as residents have complained about the companies' service quality and the payment system. Urbaser and FCC incurred municipal fines of LE 12 million (US$2 million) in response to citizens' complaints about irregular waste collection operations and inadequate street cleaning.

In February 2003, hundreds of Zabaleen took to the streets of Giza to campaign against the influx of foreign companies. As one journalist explained, 'Although the contracts were signed over six months ago, many of the Zabaleen in Giza were not aware of this development affecting their livelihood' (Rashed, 2003). However, in Cairo, the Zabaleen were kept better informed of the privatisation plans, with discussions being held with officials and government representatives and multinational companies. Nevertheless the Zabaleen were dissatisfied with the negotiations as a result of limited employment opportunities and low payment fees.

According to the official development strategy, the privatisation of waste management services was regarded as fundamental to wider government plans for the rehabilitation of medieval Cairo (Fahmi and Sutton, 2006). The objectives of the rehabilitation programme tended to favour tourism-orientated projects, while ignoring the local population's interests, through the proposed removal of informal Zabaleen settlements on Muqattam mountain, and through the

Figure 9.4: Egyptian waste management company (International Environmental Services)

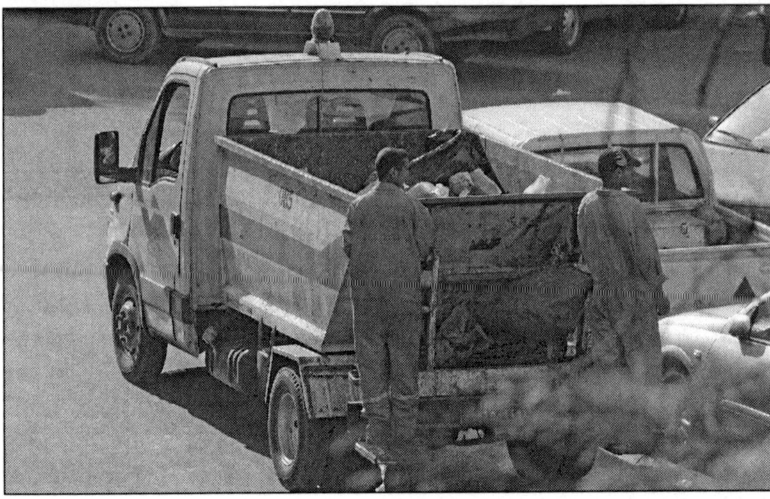

future evacuation of the nearby Eastern Cemetery's tomb dwellers and shanty-town buildings (Sutton and Fahmi, 2002a, 2002b; Fahmi and Sutton, 2003). It could be argued that the privatisation plan and eviction proposals were linked to the 1990s International Monetary Fund (IMF) Economic Reform and Structural Adjustment Programme (ERSAP) which embraced The World Bank's main economic strategies, particularly free market enterprise, currency devaluation, privatisation of state assets and public services, including waste management, reducing public spending and eradicating subsidies for low-income consumers.

More significantly, to improve living conditions for the people of Muqattam and neighbouring communities such as Manshiet Nasser, the Cairo governorate decided to move sections of the Zabaleen operations (waste recycling procedures, animal-rearing activities) 25km away to a 50-feddan plot (1 feddan = 1.038 acres), in Cairo's eastern desert settlement of Katameya. The suggested resettlement site was the same location where other government plans have sought to relocate both activities and people from medieval Cairo and from the eastern cemeteries.

Impact of the privatised waste management system

Recycling activities and housing conditions

Low-income Zabaleen respondents pinpointed security of tenure as a problem since most of them had no official documents to prove their ownership of the buildings, thus facing possible eviction, with minimal compensation. Nevertheless, the issue of compensation was raised in terms of who would be eligible, with questions as to whether there would be enough replacement housing, where it would be located and whether it would be accessible to employment and to services such as education and health centres. The situation was more stressful for those low-income Zabaleen who had set up small-scale recycling enterprises in the area, as they feared losing their source of livelihood and traditional economic activity. They were reluctant to agree to the local authority's proposed future relocation plans and to 'regularizing location of their recycling enterprises in the new areas' (Fahmi and Sutton, 2006: 823). Such a regularisation process usually involves a complex procedure full of bureaucratic delays and quite considerable expense (Sutton and Fahmi, 2002b). While they sought assistance and legal advice from local NGOs, they called for a sustained campaign in support of their case, particularly as they anticipated that they would eventually be evicted from the Zabaleen settlements in Muqattam.

Notwithstanding the relatively degrading residential environmental conditions within the settlement, plans to relocate small-scale recycling activities caused anxiety over the future, as expressed in the local narratives.

> 'If I am forced to move my work to the desert and leave my wife and daughters to travel 25km away from home, then I will stop collecting Cairo's rubbish. I start working at 4am, driving into Cairo, to collect household waste back to Muqattam settlement. Women then engage in the recycling process, sorting out the waste, picking out items (plastic, wood, glass and paper) that can be recycled and later sold.' (interviews, 2004)

> 'My family earns about LE 500 a month. But moving to Katameya will cost more in transportation. This has been our home for many years now. We have grown up, worked and raised families here. We would like to improve our conditions and to be provided with new equipment and new technologies.' (interviews, 2004)

> 'If it was not for us, how much more rubbish do you think there would be in the city? It seems the decision has already been made. There are not many alternatives for us. But I don't want to move anymore. We have already been

> forced to move many times in the past. What will happen in another 30 years? Cairo may continue to grow and then we will be forced to move once more.' (interviews, 2004)

Community livelihood and social cohesion

The five interviewed community representatives of Gammiya expressed dissatisfaction as a result of their lack of involvement in the initial launching stages of the waste restructuring project. They emphasised that their sociopolitical influence would have been instrumental in developing local awareness, among Zabaleen, of the objectives of the privatisation plans. While community leaders were initially interested in the project in terms of creating urban development potential, they suggested a six-month-long trial to ascertain the possible damage to the local economy as a result of the relocation of recycling activities, which most Zabaleen were opposed to.

Community leaders were also anxious about the Zabaleen's fate as a consequence of the privatisation plan that would disrupt the economic structure, social ties and community networks in the area. They expressed a pertinent need to find employment for the Zabaleen whose only skills were waste-related, with these being highly labour-intensive activities in which whole families were involved. The Gammiya representatives proposed a poverty alleviation programme that aimed to inform and convince official government policy and practice to reverse their decision to evict and move the Zabaleen.

Political achievement

Officials at the CCBA regarded the Zabaleen's indigenous methods of waste collection as unhygienic, with the new system separately collecting industrial, medical and household waste. CCBA officials were optimistic about the prospects of investors and businesspeople establishing 10-12 new recycling facilities in Cairo's eastern fringes. While the Zabaleen had previously recycled some 80 per cent of the waste collected, foreign companies would be required to recycle only 20 per cent, with the remainder going into a new landfill site. The Zabaleen would continue collecting waste, but they would be working for foreign companies that would also be responsible for street sweeping and for the placement of rubbish bins. An official member of staff at CCBA declared:

> 'We already have a factory operating in the Al-Salam district [Cairo's north western fringes] and are in the process of building a LE 4 million factory that will turn 50 tonnes of waste into compost daily. Three factories are under construction in Katameya desert [Cairo's eastern fringes] on an area of 25 feddan. Cairo's waste, being particularly "rich," provides great potentials for the production of high quality compost. Rather than burying the waste underground as we do now, we will be putting it to profitable use while also cleaning up the streets of Cairo.' (interviews, 2004)

Local Cairene householders, while initially enthusiastic about environmental improvements within their neighbourhoods following the restructuring of waste management, were sceptical about the direct economic benefits they might gain from the privatisation project. Instead, they preferred to continue dealing directly with the rubbish collectors, rejecting the government's plans to have them pay extra fees for services provided by multinational companies. However, local Cairene inhabitants, especially those living in slums and shanty-towns, complained more about their municipalities' failure to collect rubbish from their homes than about where the government chose to dispose of the waste. Cairo's households would be expected to pay for privatised waste collection through a monthly rate based on their electricity bill. Objections to this method of charging were expressed by Cairo's households that preferred to maintain the traditional system of relying on the Zabaleen for waste collection. In response, the High Administrative Court produced a verdict, in 2004, nullifying such extra monthly payment imposed on households, regarding it as illegal and unconstitutional.

Technical improvement

While advocating the turning of waste into compost, a leading staff member of the waste management programme at the EEAA, stressed:

> 'The recycling facilities are important because of the need to maintain a clean environment, rather than for making money. If the recycling facilities are aimed at maximising profits, then they are unlikely to be interested in the rubbish of the poor. Sixty per cent of the rubbish can be turned into compost, but the remaining 40 per cent cannot. This will be a particularly acute problem when facilities are set up

> in Upper Egypt. Where are they going to find the markets for recycled products, such as plastic, metal and paper?' (interviews, 2004)

Furthermore, representatives from AMA (the Italian company responsible for Cairo North, an area covering two million inhabitants and approximately 400,000 households) claimed that they planned to hire and train about 2,500 Zabaleen. A staff member at AMA asserted:

> 'It is our strategy to employ the local Zabaleen. We want to avoid conflict, and this satisfies the social component of our contract. We want to promote them to be up to international standards. Recyclers will still be able to go to landfills and take what they want, before the rubbish is buried. In the landfill, you'll get hotel waste that might be 100 per cent recyclable. So I think the average recovery rate might be 50 per cent.' (interviews, 2004)

Yet despite the benefits promised under foreign management, and while company sources mentioned salaries ranging between LE 300 to LE 450 per month, some Zabaleen claimed that salaries on offer were actually much lower (LE 150 per month). One rubbish collector and sorter with eight children gave similar figures:

> 'I earn LE 10 a day compared with the LE 5 a day offered by the foreign contractors. It appears that the companies realised that keeping the Zabaleen out of the system completely was not an option if they wanted to get the job of waste disposal done. Instead foreign companies have started hiring the Zabaleen as subcontractors paying them LE 0.85 for each apartment from which they collect rubbish.' (interviews, 2004)

While less than their previous collection fee of LE 3, this new arrangement would give them access to rubbish for recycling. However, the Zabaleen claimed that they made 90 per cent of their income from recycling the rubbish rather than from the collection fee.

Community empowerment and networking

Respondents at the local NGO CID expressed reservations concerning the impact of the privatisation of waste services on the Muqattam

Zabaleen community, and the role played by large international waste collection companies. Members of CID were strong opponents to the decision to force the 27,000 Muqattam workers to relocate their recycling operations (Kamel, 2003). While a leading member at CID appreciated the government's desire to keep the city clean, it was felt that the authorities should also protect the Zabaleen:

> 'The Zabaleen are facing a real crisis. The authorities need to look at the effects their decision could have on local income, employment, economic growth, trade, manufacturing and environmental conditions. I would like to see the operations of the Zabaleen formalised and given a fair chance to use new recycling technologies. The idea of moving them to the desert and squeezing them further out of their trade is not right.... These contracts are costing the city big money. Why not spend just 10 per cent of such a budget to upgrade the Zabaleen system? It's a catastrophe. Overnight, 50,000 people could be out of their jobs.' (interviews, 2004)

Several options for integrating the Zabaleen into the international companies' contracts were explored during interviews with staff members at CID, raising the issue of local–global confrontation and the possible contribution of a public–private partnership. The Zabaleen could act as subcontractors to implement a 'segregation system', dividing organic and non-organic waste. They could continue to collect household waste while multinational companies would handle medical, industrial waste and landfill management. Despite such suggestions, recent developments have demonstrated the possibility that such a fruitful local–global partnership is unlikely. Instead, international companies favoured training the Zabaleen as waged employees while also allowing them to search landfill sites for organic waste for their pig-rearing activities.

Environmental awareness

Since 1984, the local NGO APE has been working with the Zabaleen, integrating literacy and health services with income-generating activities related to paper recycling units and to an organic composting plant (APE, 1993). A degree of antagonism emerged between the APE and the Gammiya, with the latter being criticised as representing only privileged families and failing to promote the interests of the poorest rubbish collectors. Such conflict was further aggravated when APE asserted that separating Zabaleen's homes from waste and animals could improve environmental conditions within the settlement, thus expressing support for the plan to transfer waste services to Katameya. It is anticipated that APE is more likely to act alongside both government agencies and the big companies in setting up and administering new recycling activities at a local level, with the Zabaleen being engaged as waged labourers. One affiliated member at the organisation stated:

> 'It's the best idea available. There is no reason why it won't work. I don't know why people are complaining. It will improve living conditions for everyone, especially women. I understand there is opposition now, but I'm sure in time the people of Muqattam will understand the benefits the government's move will have for them.' (interviews, 2004)

Swine flu pandemic and the slaughtering of the Zabaleen's pigs

The 2009 H1N1 'swine flu' pandemic fortunately proved not to be the disaster that had been predicted, except for those concerned with Mexico's tourist industry or with Cairo's waste recycling. The Zabaleen saw their main processor of organic waste, namely, their herds of pigs, slaughtered by the Egyptian government, ostensibly on health grounds. Despite the general agreement that swine flu was not transmitted from pigs to humans, but rather directly from one person to another, the Egyptian government ordered the slaughter of up to 300,000 pigs. Later a post-facto justification was made on the grounds that a combined bird flu and swine flu outbreak, following mutation, would have endangered Egypt's population.

The Egyptian Agricultural Ministry ordered the slaughter in April 2009, and by doing so, imperilled the livelihood of about 70,000 Zabaleen families. The reported number of pigs slaughtered varied from 190,000 to 300,000, with the higher figure being most frequently quoted. Governmental health officials declared that "It has been decided to immediately start slaughtering all the pigs in Egypt using the full capacity of the country's slaughterhouses", in response to the swine flu. The government regarded the plan of culling 300,000 pigs as a judicious precaution to calm fears of the imminent pandemic. Accordingly the Zabaleen were sceptical about such a decision, as poor rubbish collectors expressed their concerns that the slaughter was just the beginning, and that the government was plotting to remove the 'Garbage City' and relocate the Zabaleen (Fahmi and Sutton, 2010).

Besides selling paper, plastic and homemade handicrafts from recycled waste, pigs were the main source of income for the Zabaleen. Hitherto, the Zabaleen claimed to collect 6,000 tonnes of waste a day, of which 60 per cent was food and organic waste that their pigs consumed. Every six months, the waste collectors sold five to fifteen adult pigs to a trader for LE 7 per kilogram. The trader then took the pigs to the slaughterhouse, where a kilogram was sold for LE 30-35. The waste collectors could earn around LE 450 per pig.

Such governmental action forced all pork processors and retail outlets to close. Bereft of their herds of pigs, the Zabaleen stopped collecting organic waste, leaving piles of such waste in streets and other public places. This led to rotting piles of food blighting the streets in middle-class neighbourhoods such as Heliopolis, as well as in poorer districts such as Imbaba. The threat of swine flu was replaced by the threat of typhus. The Food and Agriculture Organisation of the United Nations (FAO) called Egypt's action a mistake while no Egyptian was reported as falling ill with swine flu before the slaughter; since then, 891 cases have been reported, with two deaths (Fahmi and Sutton, 2010).

There were protest riots on the part of some Zabaleen in their district of Manshiet Nasser-Muqattam. Signs of malnutrition reportedly appeared among Zabaleen children as pork had been a major source of protein for them. The reason for the slaughter of the pigs changed over time as health officials worldwide claimed that the flu virus was not passed on directly by pigs. The government then claimed that the cull was no longer about the flu threat, but about belatedly cleaning up the Zabaleen's crowded, filthy neighbourhood.

Government compensation was paid, but former meat processors would pay the Zabaleen US$200 per pig. The government has offered LE 250 as compensation for an adult pig, LE 100 for a male pig, and LE 50 for a piglet. A month later the Minister of Agriculture decided to keep 1,000 pigs and breed them in specialised governmental farms near 15th of May City (an industrial area outside Cairo), to preserve the origins of the Egyptian stock, while the pigs' owners would be compensated financially. It is uncertain whether the Zabaleen will have an opportunity to begin pig breeding again.

As well as the consequence that many rubbish collectors stopped collecting organic waste, International Environmental Services (IES) suspended operations in Giza governorate for a few months, from April 2009 until September 2009, as a result of a financial dispute with the municipality. This contributed to the piling up of rubbish, with organic waste being a source of infectious disease. Some rubbish collectors also abandoned the recycling business, because without pigs, the tedious work of sorting through paper, cans and bottles was economically unfeasible. According to one rubbish collector who lost his pigs: "I have lost everything. The government paid me between LE 50 and LE 250 for each pig I lost, depending on its size, while meat processors would have given me as much as LE 1,000" (interviews, 2009).

The adverse effect of the slaughtering of the pigs on the Zabaleen's livelihoods might be part of the ongoing gentrification of the 'Garbage City' for land speculation and the taking over of their recycling economy by entrepreneurial businesses investing in Cairo's contested waste. Again, probably a post-facto justification, the *Al-Ahram* newspaper has suggested that a modern-day alternative to pig rearing based on recycled rubbish would be to convert organic waste into ethanol, as already occurs in Brazil, the US and Canada. Employing such a 'biomass process' one tonne of raw unsorted waste, with 75 per cent organic composition, would yield about 50 gallons of ethanol, which could be used as an additive to gasoline to increase its octane composition and to lower pollution from vehicles. It is claimed that this would be price-competitive as well as a recycling solution (Mitwally, 2009). This latest serious threat to Cairo's Zabaleen community only serves to compound earlier problems stemming from moves to bring in multinational waste contractors and from policies aiming to relocate waste-processing activities to remoter desert locations to the east of Cairo (Fahmi and Sutton, 2006).

Future of privatised waste management

Kamel (2003) has suggested several options for integrating the Zabaleen into the international companies' contracts. Transfer stations could be established where a major proportion of the non-organic waste could be recovered and directed to existing traders. The Zabaleen could continue to collect household waste from high-income areas on a daily, door-to-door basis, and then pass the residual waste on, after recycling, to the big companies. The Zabaleen could receive inorganic waste from the companies as an input to their recycling businesses, and could contract for selected waste, such as paper from print shops. Small community-based composting facilities could be established. The Zabaleen could pool their financial assets such as trucks and workshops. And their nationwide trading network in recycled waste could be connected to the formal sector of the solid waste economy. The traditional informal Zabaleen system could therefore be integrated into the new privatised large-scale waste collection system to the mutual benefit of both sides of the operation. However, one wonders whether in Cairo the 'private' element of the public–private partnership would include or exclude the Zabaleen. Would the new situation merely be one in which the Zabaleen work as waged labourers for the international companies? The possible contribution of a public–private partnership can be mooted in this local–global confrontation. This would represent dependency rather than partnership.

Despite suggestions made by some NGOs such as CID that the Zabaleen could continue pig rearing while collecting rubbish, sorting it, and then selling it to the international companies for recycling at facilities in Cairo's eastern fringes, developments have demonstrated this possibility as unlikely. As international expertise meets local practice, a situation of confrontation is more likely than partnership, and the NGOs are likely to have a new role under these changed circumstances. The relocation of the sorting activities will disrupt the Zabaleen's economic sustainability, particularly in pig rearing. Indeed, the whole Zabaleen recycling industry is likely to modify its links with *wahiya* contractors and with local NGOs involved in the area since the 1980s. These include APE's paper recycling and rug-weaving activities involving female members of Zabaleen households and EQI's upgrading under The World Bank Programme and its establishment of small-scale enterprises as part of ZEDP. While the Zabaleen are facing a dramatic and disruptive situation, the *wahiya* and these local NGOs can be expected to develop new mechanisms for cooperation with the international companies and with their recycling businesses relocated to eastern Cairo's urban fringes.

These expectations of collaboration between the NGOs, the *wahiya* and the international companies are based on APE's positive reaction to the privatisation plans and to the claimed possibility of improving the Zabaleen's livelihoods. Further support for this opinion comes from EQI's reports on the Zabaleen's inability to shift from being dependent on the professional assistance provided by The World Bank and various foreign funding agencies since the launch of the 1980s upgrading programme (Volpi, 1996; EQI, 1982). The EQI's reports also raise the question of the failure of NGOs to empower the local Zabaleen through community initiatives since the 1980s (Alamazani, 2011). They have also failed to assist the Zabaleen in building channels of communication with government agencies. Instead there have been conflicts with the Gammiya and with community leaders regarding recycling activities. The NGOs have not succeeded in creating any powerful grassroots lobbying to present the Zabaleen's case to public opinion as a mechanism to confront recent governmental privatisation plans. It would appear that their business interests now prevail over the NGOs' earlier role of promoting the Zabaleen community.

The slow progress of the new waste management system has not only been attributed to the Zabaleen's determination to preserve their source of livelihood (supported by NGOs such as CID), but also to households' negative attitudes towards the multinationals' performance. Officials at CCBA seemed to neglect the scale aspect of the proposed changes; namely, that the large companies could not collect from narrow streets in low-income areas as their mechanised equipment was too large. The companies required residents to take their waste to central collection points, whereas the Zabaleen were able to collect waste from individual houses, even if located in narrow alleyways. Consequently, some companies hired the Zabaleen to collect waste in those areas. Since December 2004, many residents, who were accustomed to the Zabaleen's door-to-door services, preferred to rely on the traditional waste collection service, thus refusing to deposit their wastes in the companies' rubbish bins. Multinational waste management operations therefore face an ambiguous future. Whereas Onyx in Alexandra, and AMA in Cairo, have both managed to achieve relative success in their waste management operations, other companies (such as Enser and FCC) have halted their operations and even terminated their contracts.

Conclusion

Despite official restrictions on their activities, the Zabaleen have continued to collect Cairo's waste, alongside the operations of some multinational companies and the local municipality, an indication of ongoing competition for Cairo's daily waste. The Zabaleen work throughout the day in shifts as each group sorts out the rubbish on site into piles of cardboard, glass and plastic for collection later on (via donkey carts, mini-cabs and small trucks, as well as on foot). The government should have supported the Zabaleen in improving their system, while establishing official waste management operations in less serviced and more remote areas. A more preferable outcome for the Zabaleen would have been to recognise them as stakeholders in the waste management system. This scenario would have involved a hybrid corporate micro-enterprise service, with the Zabaleen's recycling methods being integrated into the formal waste management system, and with multinational companies focusing on establishing and maintaining landfill sites and waste treatment plants.

The Zabaleen's integration into the formal waste management system will depend on the outcome of the current state of upheaval within Cairo and Egypt since the 2011 uprising. Similar causes that have perpetuated the Zabaleen's situation also motivated the post-2011 uprising. Political repression, lack of democratic freedom and unsatisfactory neoliberal economic policy reform, which did not adequately resolve inflation, poverty and high unemployment rates, should all be taken into consideration when assessing the Zabaleen's future. However, dispossessed societal groups such as the Zabaleen may be more adequately equipped to deal with the post-2011 uprising uncertainties and difficulties that have characterised their existence for decades.

In addition, behind the declared official rationalisation for the eviction proposals in terms of 'improving the environment' lies a wider but hidden agenda in terms of securing access to land for urban development projects and land speculation activities. This is mainly attributed to two factors. On the one hand, the 'Garbage City' within Muqattam mountain's lower plateau provides urban investment opportunities as a result of its geographical proximity to Cairo's historical quarters and its tourist-orientated urban rehabilitation projects. On the other hand, Muqattam City, located on the mountain's upper plateau, represents both a powerful pressure group and an urban development model to the detriment of the waste recyclers. This is noted in the proposed planning of a luxury residential gated community project (Uptown Cairo) by the Dubai-based Emaar property development company (Fahmi and Sutton, 2006).

This study has identified the need for local government's support for community initiatives to develop small-scale recycling enterprises and income-generating activities for the Zabaleen who are threatened with relocation. This could be done through mutual self-help, and through soft loans, subsidies and technical support to improve, rebuild or expand their new homes. In the case of the Zabaleen's proposed eviction, there is a need to tackle problems in the new settlements of inadequate provision of water supply, sanitation and drainage. Any reorganisation of the collection and disposal of waste should be in partnership with the different stakeholders, from relocatees to community leaders, NGOs, local authorities and other agencies. Local NGOs with a strong commitment to participation tend to keep costs down while avoiding the reinforcement of patronage, thus creating less dependency among relocated local communities.

In conclusion, this study advocates radical policy action and collaborative planning for consolidating bottom-up urban governance. There is a need to strengthen the urban poor's capacity to negotiate with local authorities for security of land tenure and legal recognition of the 'Garbage City'. Partnership between community-based groups, NGOs, local authorities and planners would support the urban poor's sustainable initiatives to improve their housing standards and basic services, and to develop small-scale enterprises and affordable means of transport.

References

Alamazani, K. (2011) 'Egypt – The Zabbaleen Environmental Development Program (ZEDP)', *Informal Waste Pickers and Recyclers (IWPAR), Towards social inclusion and protection of informal waste pickers and recyclers, Best Practices No 1* (www.iwpar.org/id-1-egypt-the-zabaleen.html).

APE (Association for the Protection of the Environment) (1993) 'Proposal for upgrading and expansion of the Zabbaleen paper project', Unpublished document, Cairo: Cairo Governorate.

Assaad, M. and Garas, N. (1994) 'Experiments in community development in a Zabbaleen settlement', *Cairo Papers in Social Science*, vol 16, no 4, Cairo: The American University in Cairo.

EQI (Environmental Quality International) (1982) *Strategies for upgrading solid waste management in Cairo: Policies and programs*, Report No 5, Solid waste component: First Egypt Urban Development Project, Cairo: EQI.

Fahmi, W. (2005) 'The impact of privatization of solid waste management on the Zabaleen garbage collectors of Cairo', *Environment and Urbanization*, vol 17, no 2, pp 155-70.

Fahmi, W. and Sutton, K. (2003) 'Reviving historical Cairo through pedestrianisation: The Al-Azhar street axis', *International Development Planning Review*, vol 25, no 4, pp 407-31.

Fahmi, W. and Sutton, K. (2006) 'Cairo's Zabaleen garbage recyclers: Multinationals' takeover and state relocation plans', *Habitat International*, vol 30, no 4, pp 809-37.

Fahmi, W. and Sutton, K. (2010) 'Cairo's contested garbage: Sustainable solid waste management and the Zabaleen's right to the city', *Sustainability*, no 2, pp 1765-83.

Golia, M. (2004) *Cairo: City of sand*, London: Reaktion Books.

Kamel, L. (2003) 'Integrating local community-based waste management into international contracting', Paper No 31, CWG Workshop, Dar El Salaam, Tanzania, 9-14 March.

Mitwally, E. (2009) 'Conversion of domestic solid waste into Ethanol', *Al-Ahram Weekly Online*, 22-28 October (http://weekly.ahram.org.eg/2009/969/sc71.htm).

Motaal, D.A. (1996) 'Reconstructing development: Women of the Muqattam Zabbalinsettlement', *Cairo Paper in Social Science*, vol 19, no 4, pp 59-110, Cairo: The American University in Cairo.

Nzeadlibe, T.C. (2009) 'Solid waste reforms and informal recycling in Enugu urban area', *Habitat International*, vol 33, no 1, pp 93-9.

Rashed, D. (2003) 'Trashed lives', *Al-Ahram Weekly Online*, no 624, 6-12 February (http://weekly.ahram.org.eg/2003/624/fe1.htm).

Sutton, K. and Fahmi, W. (2002a) 'The rehabilitation of old Cairo', *Habitat International*, vol 26, no 1, pp 73-93.

Sutton, K. and Fahmi, W. (2002b) 'Cairo's "cities of the dead": The myths, problems, and future of a unique squatter settlement', *The Arab World Geographer*, vol 5, no 1, pp 1-21.

Vincentian Missionaries (1998) 'The Payatas environmental development programme: Microenterprise promotion and involvement in solid waste management in Quezon City', *Environment and Urbanization*, vol 10, no 2, pp 55-68.

Visser, M. and Theron, J. (2009) *Waste not: Externalisation and the movement of waste in Cape Town*, Institute for Poverty, Land and Agrarian Studies (PLAAS) Working Paper 12, Cape Town: Institute for Poverty, Land and Agrarian Studies.

Volpi, E. (1996) 'The Zabbalin community of Muqattam: Community organization and development among the Zabbalin of Muqattam', *Cairo Papers in Social Science*, vol 19, no 4, pp 8-64.

TEN

Ecomodern discourse and localised narratives: waste policy, community mobilisation and governmentality in Ireland

Liam Leonard

Introduction

When examining issues in Irish waste management, many competing tensions begin to surface. These include tensions between the policy discourse of ecological modernisation and the local narratives by which communities relate to their environment. Furthermore, tensions can be detected between the demands of international bodies such as the European Union (EU), who demand efficient and regulated waste policies, and the more economically derived focus of the Irish state. The following analysis of Irish waste management explores the dichotomies between the discourse and narrative that surrounds this contested issue.

The chapter is divided into five main sections and a conclusion. The first section examines the *narratives* that underpin much of the debates about communities and their environments in the Irish case. The second section outlines the concept of ecological modernisation as it has developed in *governance* since the late 1990s. The third examines the emergence of the Irish state's *regional waste plans* introduced in the 1990s. The plans were significant due to their attempt to create commodified waste pathways across a number of regions in Ireland. The fourth section analyses the *millennium report* on Ireland's environment (Environmental Protection Agency, 2000). The fifth section looks at the *community response* to these waste plans, along with the subsequent mobilisation of campaigns of resistance to the inclusion of incineration as an option for waste management in the Irish case. The chapter concludes with a discussion about issues of governmentality and waste in Ireland's regions.

The chapter also examines the urban and the rural, as there is less of a divide between these two elements in Irish society than in other European states, and domestic waste flows and salient discourses on the subject impinge on both sectors in an overlapping manner. Table 10.1, based on the discursive framing analysis in the initial research for Leonard (2005, 2006), illustrates the parameters of this contested issue by separating it into constituent frames and outcomes, be they political, cultural, social, legal, institutional, economic or scientific. Table 10.1 locates the impacts and outcomes of community mobilisations in environmental disputes involving the Irish state, multinationals and the EU.

Narratives: socioenvironmental narratives and the community

This form of rural ecocentricism can be understood through an examination of 'rural sentiment' (Leonard, 2006). This concept has emerged from an analysis of existing studies of local environmentalism and rural change in the Irish case. Initial accounts of 'rural fundamentalism' (Commons, 1996, p 30) provide a basis for an understanding of the resistance to state-sponsored rural development projects as Irish agriculture has become more industrialised in recent years. Resistance to perceived interference from the state or Europe derives from a localised sense of mutual dependency and embeddedness within the local hinterlands of rural Ireland. As modernisation and economic growth occurred, a concept of 'rural discourse' has been forwarded to describe local responses to the location of multinational factories in rural areas (Peace, 1997, pp 10-22).

However, this discourse was in itself a representation of a primordial or visceral 'rural sentiment' (Leonard, 2006, 2008) that became manifest at times of societal discord in rural Ireland. Through time, this underlying sentiment has become a discourse of fundamentalism in the face of external threats to local communities or landscapes that are etched within the subconscious of rural dwellers. Part of the process of contestation in waste disputes has involved calls to protect the landscape, hills and coastline of the west of Ireland that is, in many ways, a living entity to its inhabitants, in a manner that has parallels with aboriginal tribes globally.

Table 10.1: A discursive framing analysis of Irish environmental movements

Frame	Type of campaign	Type of protest/ tactics	Framing outcome	Political outcome
Political	Concerns for democratic deficit and party support/ opposition; local political allies, national political allies Exploiting political opportunities, electoral leverage	Local alliances, national alliances, global alliances, embedded advocate, framing issues, political opportunities	Mobilisation of grievance consensus at local and national level; heightened awareness of environmental issues and democratic deficit	Increased political access and leverage
Social	NIMBYism, grassroots alternative energies among new middle-class professionals, working class	Populism supported or opposed by local interests, health risks, marches, demonstrations	Evolving from NIMBYism into wider movement	Increased politicisation of civil society
Cultural	Rural discourse/eco-feminist discourse, moral discourse/religions, use of interest-led expertise, nationalist discourse	External advocate, mobilised resources, cultural and heritage frames, media and celebrity advocacy	More expansive media coverage; discursive interpretations of culture and heritage	Enhanced sociopolitical and cultural discourse
Legal	Oral hearing, High Court, European Court	Legal challenges to policy or projects	Establishing precedents or overturning laws or policy	Redefined policy agendas; changes to legal framework
Institutional/ agencies	EU – UN – sustainable development, local authority support or opposition, to the state, heritage of planning bodies	Legal campaigns, expertise advocacy, institutional allies, political allies	Enhanced understanding of overall issue from grassroots grievance to institutional frameworks	Reinforced linkages between institutional sector and community
Economic	Pre-growth – pollution, resource protection, post-growth infrastructural development	Anti-multinational, anti-state, opposition to sitings	Establishing grievance over costs and location of projects	Projects delayed or shelved
Scientific	Global networks	Interest-led advocacy	Counter-arguments to scientific viewpoints presented	State and industrial science challenged

Source: After Leonard (2005, 2006)

The transition from a traditional agrarian society into an urbanised modern economy has not been without its difficulties for some sections of Ireland's rural population. A primary area of contention that has emerged is the development of state and industrial infrastructures such as power plants, incinerators and road networks. Alongside these issues, local communities have been faced with changing sociocultural values that appear to be outside of their control. Furthermore, the state's move away from traditional rural industries such as agriculture and tourism in favour of multinational-led development has led to many rural dwellers questioning the type of society which is emerging in Ireland. In addition, major industrial and infrastructural developments have threatened local environments.

For many the changes that have occurred in rural Ireland over the last half century have mirrored a disengagement from the traditional patterns of life that had embedded a set of values and practices which allowed rural communities to coexist with their surrounding environment. In the era of globalised production, local production for local markets has come to be dismissed as small-minded thinking. The damage caused to local interactions between communities and hinterlands has been significant.

One response to this loss of local identity was the concept of 'rural development' (Leonard 2006, 2008) which involved community-based initiatives reinvigorating local discourse in the face of outside challenges, both culturally and environmentally speaking. A combination of grievances relating to depopulation, unemployment and neglect of rural regions has provided successive environmental campaigns with a groundswell of dissent to facilitate 'mobilisation' processes against multinationals or the political establishment. When combined with the renewed confidence achieved by new middle-class figures bolstered by expertise on rural rejuvenation programmes learned during migrant experiences abroad, a significant form of rural-based resistance has emerged. This fundamental response has come to be articulated around 'defence of space' types of territorial campaigns involving the imposition of industrial plants or infrastructural projects.

The underlying themes of populist rural discourse are in themselves sufficient for the development of rural attitudes in the face of ecological degradation in the regions. However, it is felt that a discourse could only emerge from something more intrinsically held in the collective consciousness of a community, the basis of identities formed in an area over centuries and passed down among indigenous peoples. Ultimately, it is this embedded sentiment that becomes ignited, leading to any subsequent discourse of community protest, as the 'unifying ether' (Leonard, 2006, 2008) of ecological capital is sparked into the flames of collective action.

The backdrop to the emergence of environmental disputes in Ireland has been the development of a form of community politics that has its basis in a rural identity that is embedded in Irish society. One result of this has been a growth of an identity-based community politics that challenges industrial policies and projects in the regions. This form of externalised community expression has taken shape in spite of the dependent nature of the industrialisation policies of the state, and illustrates a rural mindset that holds self-sufficiency and local wisdom drawn from interaction with the hinterland in higher regard than the conventional wisdom of the representatives of politics or industry.

Governance: ecological modernisation and the state

The conceptual basis for key turning points in the state's waste management policy is located within the parameters of an ecological modernisation approach (see also McDonagh et al, 2009). Ecological modernisation is an alternative conceptual approach to what were previously seen as problems with the 'end-of-pipe' solutions. Any costs were shown to be beneficial, as they would outweigh the future costs of repairing the damage caused by pollution. At a policy level, ecological modernisation has been used to help forge new and coordinated approaches to what were previously seen as problems facing the differing strata of bureaucracy. The state's policy shift on waste, from a reliance on landfill to a strategy informed by the EU's 'waste hierarchy', would provide many of the political opportunities for campaigners, and became a key feature of the waste dispute in Ireland. Rootes (1994, pp 15-19) argues that the conditions surrounding institutional arrangements are 'contingent and temporary', creating access to political opportunities for challengers when these institutional arrangements are changed. In the Irish case, the state has attempted to introduce a more 'stable' arrangement in relation to waste management, through institutional and policy responses. The waste crisis should be understood in the context of the increase in generated waste during the Irish period of economic growth, which was reported at an average of 10.5 per cent per annum (Environmental Protection Agency, 2003, p 13).

By creating policies to protect the environment and to promote waste management practices, the state attempted to change the behaviour of the public, corporate and municipal sectors, all of which had become over-reliant on the use of landfill sites. In some ways, the policy agenda introduced by the state to deal with the demands of the EU or concerned communities could be described as 'a blunt instrument' (Roberts, 2004, p 156) to force through regulations that dealt with obligations on the one hand, while maintaining the focus on 'economic growth' on the other. Concerned communities have challenged the state's choice of incineration as a preferred option due to perceived 'health risks'. These contradictions would emerge in the wake of the state's attempts to create a policy framework to deal with the waste issue. The technocratic centralisation of 'top-down' decision-making powers on waste management itself has created opportunities for challenges to incineration and the need for local politicians to support 'bottom-up' pressure. And by omitting any discussion of the potential health risks posed by incineration, the state was left vulnerable to the challenger's contention that incinerators in other states have created health problems in their vicinities.

Emergence of the Irish state's regional waste plans

The state established the Irish Environmental Protection Agency in 1992 to deal with environmental problems in general. Throughout the 1990s a number of Acts and policy documents were created in response to the waste crisis. These policy initiatives included the Waste Management Act 1996, the 1998 waste policy statement (Government of Ireland, 1998), the Agency's 2000 millennium report (Environmental Protection Authority, 2000) and the regional waste plans, incorporating regions such as Dublin, the South East, Galway, Limerick, the North East and the Midlands. All of these areas were to include a municipal incinerator as part of their waste management plan. The establishment of the Environmental Protection Agency was seen as a progressive initiative by the state. However, the Agency has also been criticised as not being independent from the influence of the industrialisation imperative of the state. The state then promoted environmentally progressive business practices, moving from 'end-of-pipe' solutions to a reorganisation of industrial and environmental policy, now combined in overall sustainable practices throughout the manufacturing process. While the intent of EU environmental policy is clear, non-compliant or environmentally 'laggard' member-states have continued to attract direct foreign investment from US multinationals, with EU directives on environmental regulation reduced to a secondary consideration.

By 2000, Ireland had implemented the European Community strategy for waste management that included an overall hierarchical structure for dealing with waste issues. Emphasis was placed primarily on waste prevention, recycling and reuse. The 1999 Landfill Directive (Council of the European Communities, 1999) limited the use of landfills, leaving the Irish government with no option but to search for alternatives. Local authorities had already committed to this switch to alternative waste management processes by the Waste Management Act 1996, although they did not promote such alternative processes such as recycling, preferring to present incineration as their policy of choice.

This 'top-down' approach to the regulation and disposal of waste led to an emphasis on two primary waste management options, landfilling or incineration. There was less emphasis on prevention, reduction and recycling, the EU's most favoured options, and regional community groups. In the Dublin region, targets for this objective between 1994 and 2004 were set at between '59% for recycling, 25% for thermal treatment, (incineration) and 16% for landfill' (Fingal County Council, 2002). This target was to be achieved despite the 1999 figure of up to 95 per cent of household waste being landfilled in Ireland, a figure matched only in Russia among European neighbours. Government policy on waste management was outlined in the document *Changing our ways* in 1998 (Government of Ireland, 1998), while regional waste plans were drafted at this time. The next section of this chapter examines these aspects of the government's waste management plans in detail.

The formation of the Environmental Protection Agency in 1992 provided a structured response to European Commission directives on environmental issues (Council of the European Communities, 1991). As waste management became an increasingly problematic issue, a Waste Management Act was enacted in 1996. The role of the Minister for the Environment, Local Authorities and the Environmental Protection Agency were redefined to incorporate them into a common framework for waste management policy in Ireland. The Act presented a regulatory framework for improved environmental standards in relation to the practices of prevention, minimisation and recycling. It was also devised with a structured development of a waste industry and the new technological demands of the EC's directives on waste management. The Act represented an attempt by the state to respond to the EU's waste directives, through the establishment of a policy framework that would incorporate the state, local authorities and the Environmental Protection Agency.

The responsibilities of the relevant public authorities were also set out in the Act. The core provisions of the Act include penalties of up to 10 million Euros in fines and liability for pollution clean-up costs. Agricultural, commercial or industrial obligations to prevent pollution from the design stage through the production process are dealt with in Section 28. Section 32 deals with the transportation, storage and disposal of waste. Section 39 deals with the licensing of disposal facilities and the prohibition of unlicensed disposal. Over time, illegal dumping had become a major issue, as increased dumping charges have created an illegal dumping network. The Agency was deemed responsible for waste recovery and disposal licensing, and for the management and control of hazardous waste. The Integrated Pollution Control (IPC) licensing system that was introduced by the Agency in 1992 has been maintained through the Waste Management Act 1996. The IPC approach takes a broad approach to pollution control through licensing. IPC approaches focus on all forms of pollution, seeking controls on: 'Environmentally optimal risk-reduction of pollutants with cost considerations imposed as constraint, implicitly or explicitly, on reduction effort' (Weale, 1992, p 111).

The regional, city and county local authorities have undertaken the functions of the Waste Management Act. Local authority responsibilities include a planning process to deal with non-hazardous and commercial waste, domestic waste collection, recovery and disposal, and an overall supervision of waste-related activities in their areas. The Act has placed overall power for waste management in the hands of the Minister for the Environment and Local Government.

The general provisions of the Act provide for new powers for the Environmental Protection Agency and local authorities, aimed at facilitating legislation enforcement and monitoring. Sections 14 and 15 deal with the powers of inspection and obligations towards monitoring. A framework for waste management planning is then outlined in the Act. The Agency is charged with establishing an overall hazardous waste plan in Section 26, offering recommendations on such waste to local authorities. Local authorities must prepare individual or joint waste plans for their region, and these regional waste plans are required to follow EU directives on waste management, and as such, should incorporate prevention and recovery methods. Procedures for public consultation have also been incorporated into the regional waste plan process, but submissions were only accepted as the regional plans were introduced. The Act goes on, in Section 28, to deal with regulations on waste prevention and recovery. The obligations of all waste producers such as commercial producers and consumers in industry or agricultural are outlined. Obligations are imposed to minimise or prevent waste production, through production or manufacturing processes. Sections 29 and 30 provide the Minister with regulatory powers for waste recovery. Local authorities then set environmental targets on waste recovery, in line with EU directives.

By 1998, as the provisions of the Act began to have an impact on social processes, the government introduced a wide-ranging policy statement about waste management titled *Changing our ways* (Government of Ireland, 1998). The statement reflected a common concern in government circles that waste generation was continuing to increase, while there was a lack of progress in implementing alternatives to landfill, which was deemed to be an unsophisticated approach in its current form, according to the findings from the European Environmental Agency's report *Europe's environment: The second assessment* in the Spring of 1998 (European Environment Agency, 2002). By September of that year, the Department of the Environment had launched the *Changing our ways* policy statement. The statement commenced with recognition of the fact that, 'There is an urgent need, in line with government policy and the new framework of the Waste Management Act 1996, to modernise waste management practice and secure the provision of environmentally efficient infrastructure' (Government of Ireland, 1998, p 1).

The 1998 policy statement's purpose was the provision of an overall national framework for both the local authorities and an emerging private waste industry to operate 'with confidence'. The main changes introduced through this framework include an infrastructure to cope with the regulation of the industry, and the licensing of waste management processes such as incineration, landfilling and recycling. Local authorities in Ireland are charged with taking 'a pivotal role' to effect these changes. The policy statement was presented as a continuation from other strategy documents, such as *Recycling for Ireland* (July 1994) and *Sustainable development: A strategy for Ireland* (April 1997) (Department for the Environment, 1994, 1997). The transition from policy to the adoption and implementation of waste management plans was also recognised as an area in need of attention. The policy statement spoke of the need to 'address this challenge with vision and vigour' so as 'to secure radical change ' and of 'the need to be ambitious' in relation to the implementation of waste policy (Government of Ireland, 1998, p 2). There was also recognition that Ireland needed to go 'beyond a basic compliance with national and EU legislation, incorporating best practice and resource efficiency in economic sectors' (Government of Ireland, 1998, p 2). The statement also reinforced the importance of the 'polluter pays' principle as 'fundamental' to waste management efficiency, while emphasising the importance of economies of scale that took into account the viabilities of waste strategies.

Local opposition to landfills is recognised in the statement. 'Nuisance factors' are listed as including 'odours, dust, litter, noise, rodents, insects and general unsightliness' (Government of Ireland, 1998, p 4). The future of waste management was incorporated into the parameters of the Waste Management Act 1996, in addition to a 'flexible legislative framework' (Government of Ireland, 1998, p 4). The role of the local authorities in waste management and 'a strong emphasis on public consultation' (Government of Ireland, 1998, p 4) were presented as key components for waste management strategies. The process of planning for the future should also incorporate the type of neo-corporatist arrangements envisaged under Agenda 21: 'A new approach to environmental management, involving constructive cooperation with local communities and neighbouring local authorities, and utilising the potential of the private sector to contribute in the delivery of public services' (Government of Ireland, 1998, p 4). The creation of local authority and private sector partnerships was also seen as a positive future strategy, highlighting an ideological shift from state to market-based solutions. The increased participation of the private sector in waste management was something that the policy statement also encouraged, in order to facilitate an increase in capital expenditure and investment, technological expertise, marketplace knowledge, combined with the positive effect of freeing up local authority staff and finances for use in other services. The statement went on to explore the development of a market infrastructure for recovery and recycling, including partnership approaches and investment in waste facilities. This reflected the government's faith in a technocratic and market solution to the waste issue, using incineration technology in a 'market infrastructure'.

The 2000 Environmental Protection Agency millennium report

According to the Environmental Protection Agency (2000) millennium report on Ireland's environment, nearly 80 million tonnes of waste were generated in Ireland in 1998, mostly from agricultural production. Two million tonnes of municipal waste were produced that year along with 91 million tonnes of industrial waste. This amounted to an over 100 per cent rise in waste collected by local authorities in the years between 1984 and 1998. This period also witnessed an increase of 47 per cent in the generation of industrial waste, combined with an increase of 13 per cent in hazardous waste. In addition, the Agency (2000) indicates that 2.7 million tonnes of construction and demolition waste were produced in 1998 alone, an amount which is projected to significantly increase due to the increase in construction taking place throughout Ireland.

The destination of this waste material has primarily been landfill sites, with as high as 91 per cent of Irish municipal waste being landfilled in 1998. The millennium report charts recovery rates for packaging waste at 14.8 per cent, although some progress has been made in this area during the intervening years. Industrial waste recovery improved between 1995 and 1998, rising from 12.4 to 26.6 per cent. Manufacturing recovery rates during the same period improved from

30 per cent to 51.4 per cent, according to the report, indicating some success for the Agency's emphasis on private sector partnership (2000).

Priority issues included the minimisation of waste production, in addition to attempts to 'break the link between economic growth and waste production' (Environmental Protection Agency, 2000: 58). This waste contained materials such as paper, glass, plastics, aluminium and other metals, textiles and organic waste. According to the report, Ireland differs from its EU neighbours by not having introduced incineration, a point that is seen to be at variance with the ethos of EU environmental policy: 'In the absence of incineration, landfill will continue to be the primary disposal route for household and commercial waste, despite the fact the EU policy considers landfill to be the least desirable waste management practice' (Environmental Protection Agency 2000: 58).

As recycling was the main alternative to incineration, according to community groups, the affordability and infrastructure for this process becomes crucial. Recovery rates for the purposes of recycling household and commercial waste increased from 7.8 per cent in 1995 to 9.0 per cent in 1998. A decrease from 4.3 to 3.2 per cent in household paper waste collection in the same period was due to declining household paper waste collection during this period. However, household glass collection rates improved, from 7,900 tonnes in 1995 to 14,100 tonnes in 1998. Despite these successes, the Agency acknowledged that 'material waste recycling is a volatile and uncertain business' (Environmental Protection Agency, 2000, p 58), due to fluctuation in the value of recycled waste, and to recycling rates remaining unpredictable, and market solutions remained problematic, due to prohibitive costs. The report went on to highlight again the lack of incineration in the Irish case: 'Owing to the absence of municipal waste incineration capacity in Ireland their targets have to be met by recycling alone' (2000, p 59). European Commission directives on packaging waste has called for an EU-wide approach to the recovery and recycling of glass bottles, aluminium cans and paper containers which make up packaging waste materials. Irish recovery targets aimed at a 25 per cent recovery rate for 2001, rising to a 50-65 per cent rate of recovery for 2005. The Environmental Protection Agency (2006, p 5) reported that the recycling of packaging waste stood 'at 60% recycling in 2005, achieving and exceeding the Packaging Directive target of 50% recycling by 2005'.

Industrial waste grew from 6.2 to 9.1 million tonnes from 1995 to 1998, an increase in 47 per cent, most of which was produced by the manufacturing sector. Seventy-three per cent of this industrial waste was disposed of through landfill, with 27 per cent recovered through the IPC licensing system. The 1998 figure for hazardous waste was 370,000 tonnes, up 13 per cent (Environmental Protection Agency, 2000). A total of 35.6 per cent of this hazardous waste was disposed of or recovered on site, with 11.5 per cent disposed of off-site. A further 26.9 per cent was exported. Construction waste accounted for 2.7 million tonnes, with 1.17 million tonnes of this being recovered for road fill (Environmental Protection Agency, 2000). All of these figures are indicative of the increased consumerism and construction waste, which has forced the state to search for waste management alternatives.

The next best options for waste management are recovery and reuse which, according to the millennium report, include 'recycling and energy recovery' (incineration), with the added proviso that: 'When considering the net environmental impact, this needs to be balanced against the overall cost to the environment in relation to energy usage and pollution that might arise as a result of the recovery process itself' (2000, p 65).

One such area of pollution that would stem from the recovery process is the emissions from incineration. Incineration or 'thermal treatment' is 'the subject of some debate', according to the millennium report. The absence of incineration in Ireland is in 'marked contrast to other European countries' (2000, p 67). The report indicated the state's desire to increase efficiency in waste management as part of their ecomodern approach to concepts such as energy recovery. The report further stated that: 'It appears likely that Ireland will see the introduction of thermal treatment with energy recovery for municipal waste, particularly in large urban areas' (2000, p 66).

The Agency forecast a continued increase in waste production rates due to the 'stubborn linkage' between economic growth and waste production. A link was established between the sustainability of the economy and the consumption and use for resources. The Agency adapted a sustainable waste management approach in an attempt to minimise the impact of increased waste production. As the pressures on the environment increase through waste production, infrastructural development of roads, networks and increased construction, Ireland's accelerated expansion has come under further scrutiny from environmental groups.

Community response to waste regional plans: governance and waste management disputes in Ireland

The state's six regional waste plans in Dublin, the South East, Connacht (West), the Midlands, the North East and the Mid West were conceived to provide local solutions to the waste crisis to allow 'an economy of scale' approach to the waste issue, which could deal with the dispersal population in rural areas. The Connacht draft waste management plan was prepared by consultants MC O'Sullivan, in association with COWI incineration from Denmark. It was devised as the waste management plan for the western counties of Galway, Mayo, Sligo, Leitrim and Roscommon, in addition to Galway City. The plan was prepared in accordance with the Waste Management Act 1996. Each of the relevant local authorities was presented with a waste management strategy in the Spring of 1999. This strategy recommended integrated approaches to waste management, such as recycling, biological and thermal treatment or incineration of waste, in addition to landfilling to environmental standards. The draft plan was put on public display at local authority offices for a two-month period before the plan's adoption. The power to adopt the plan rested with the elected members of the local authorities (Galway City Council, 2001).

Community campaigns achieved various degrees of political access, with differing consequences. Environmental movement activism can therefore be seen to influence policy in the context of waste infrastructure and its political governance. Three regional campaigns occurred in the 1990s and early 2000s in the Derry, Galway and Cork regions. A waste management crisis emerged as a result of increased consumption rates as economic growth was achieved in the Republic and as a post-conflict process was emerging in the north. European directives led to a shift from a traditional over-reliance on landfill, with regional waste management plans including incineration as an option for the first time. In the course of the mobilisation of networks for the anti-incinerator and 'zero waste' movements, the role of experts and advocates with international experience of similar protests, the significance of cultural capital in the mobilisation process and differences in the rural and urban campaigns became a significant feature of those campaigns. It is also interesting to note the extent to which political access was achieved by community groups originally alienated from the mainstream of politics in both jurisdictions.

Waste management issues and the broader issue of sustainable development raise issues concerning governance in contemporary societies. 'Governance' refers to the interactions between civil society and governments in issues of local politics. Effective governance includes positive political behaviours such as transparency, efficiency, openness, sustainability and accountability. Recognition of civil society actors such as community groups and environmental groups who that may have concerns about the government's waste management strategies, infrastructural projects or sustainable development in particular should be incorporated into mediation and consultation processes.

Conclusion: governmentality and waste

This chapter has examined the mobilisation and political opportunities surrounding the governance of waste in both jurisdictions in Ireland. It has demonstrated how regional campaigns with links with the global anti-incinerator and 'zero-waste' campaigns, and from the support of experts from the US and Britain, successfully challenged the Irish state's regional waste policies. As a result, this regional waste policy was negated, as communities began to inform themselves of the dangers posed by the dioxins and furans which are released into the air and food chain from incinerator emissions (Leonard, 2008). Nonetheless, there were also many positive outcomes to the community engagement with the waste issue, and regional recycling was introduced in many areas with great success. Each of the campaigns met with differing outcomes, due to the nature of the political frameworks in those jurisdictions. The three Irish case studies presented here demonstrate differing responses by social mobilisations to the state's governance of waste management.

Environmental social movements have emerged since the years of economic growth, while concerns about the effects of ecological degradation have increased. These movements have challenged concepts of industrialised growth that have dominated political thinking over recent centuries. Although environmental groups can network with one another, exchanging expertise and support, the localised focus on environmental grievances can lead to accusations of 'NIMBYism', or the 'Not In My Backyard' syndrome. NIMBYism entails local populist opposition to sitings of toxic industries or waste plants in localities or neighbourhoods. NIMBY groups frame the 'moral discourse' (Grove-White, 1993) surrounding the environmental and health risks facing communities where toxic plants are situated, and highlight the potential economic and health costs which may result from the distribution of toxic effluents and emissions. These NIMBY groups are characterised by intensive outbreaks of local activism, as public responses are galvanised in opposition to hazardous plants. Protests are used to bargain for the restoration or maintenance of collective goods such as clean air waterways.

The Discursive Event Analysis chart at the beginning of this chapter maps out the manner in which communities can influence policy on issues such as waste management, through the framing processes they undertake as part of their campaigns. Environmental organisations may be dependent on the goodwill of external agencies for other resources, such as financial contributions or favourable media coverage. In order to attract such support, environmental organisations depict themselves in a framing process that may exploit the wider sympathies of a public that may be supportive of environmental issues without wishing to become full participants in a campaign. In this way, environmental groups may exploit wider public concern for the global commons, given that shared environmental goods such as clean air or food products invoke a degree of concern across society. Accusations of NIMBYism may therefore be overcome through an incisive framing process, as environmental movements present themselves as responsible protectors of the environment. Environmental movements may undergo an 'ideological development' (Szasz, 1994, p 77), as increased professionalism, wider networks and political interaction create understandings of how environmental issues overlap at a national or global level.

Environmental movements in waste campaigns may have a shared or 'collective' interest, and pursue goals which will challenge or change institutions, without operating through the channels of formal party politics. As the institutions of the state fail to deal with the environmental grievances of communities, movements are organised around issues of local concerns. Indeed, due to the state's primary focus on infrastructural development and competitiveness, state agencies are often the target of environmental movement campaigns. If the political process is seen to be exclusive, and policy that has an ecologically harmful aspect is seen as imposed undemocratically, then movements can form to express alternative or oppositional positions. As political parties, industries and trade unions map out their policies, environmental issues may be overlooked during the planning and implementation of policies such as waste management. This can lead to civil society activity in response to perceptions of 'democratic deficit' on matters of environmental concern, as some social groups feel left out of the political arrangements based on corporatist relations. The closure on competitiveness by the state and its neo-corporatist partners in Ireland has also led to Irish environmental movements facing political closure. However, this exclusion also creates opportunities for civil society campaigns.

One result of the wider support enjoyed by environmental movements has been an increase in levels of professionalism and bureaucratic control. The role of civil society has evolved in contemporary society, as the requirement for expertise in areas such as management, media, politics and science has increased. The representation of environmental interests has also become dependent on a group's ability to frame an environmental or waste issue in a manner that attracts the public's attention, using issues such as health or ecological protection. State and corporate interests in environmental issues are being represented with a greater degree of sophistication due to public interest in environmental or waste management issues, and must be matched by increasingly sophisticated challengers. This may lead to a movement losing touch with more radical groups, and could create problems for challengers, as the authorities may exploit internal movement tensions, making success more difficult.

Local responses to a national or international environmental issue may vary in line with the availability of expertise within movement organisations. Additional factors which environmental movements must contend with include the extent to which control over environmental or development issues is centralised, the competency of the tier of government which must be dealt with, and the manner in which policies which affect local environments or communities are implemented. Perspectives on the future direction of the Irish environmental movement began to emerge during the years of growth synonymous with the 'Celtic Tiger' economy. As the contexts of environmental disputes shifted from concerns about toxic industries towards a debate about the problems of consumerism and waste in Irish society, the focus of environmental campaigns was redirected, while a debate commenced as to the future of environmental movements in Ireland. The specific nature of localised or NIMBYist environmental campaigns in Ireland led to a kind of tunnel vision for Irish environmental movements. The opportunities for bridge-building and movement cooperation were not to be seized by the disparate groups campaigning against pollution in their local communities. This networking was defined as occurring between people involved in groups, rather than through groups themselves.

The apparent disregard by authorities for community consultation in both jurisdictions in Ireland can be seen as the primary contributing factor (and political opportunity) for environmental movement responses to policy. These various movements shared certain features, and drew from similar pools of internal and external resources, as an anti-multinational and NIMBY frame in the 1970s and 1980s gave way to concerns about the negative impacts of the economic boom in the waste management policy frameworks of the 1990s and 2000s (Rootes and Leonard, 2010; Leonard, 2011).

Research over the years has demonstrated the manner in which Irish anti-incinerator campaigns were able to avail of these internal and external resources, as the shifting dynamic of political opportunities evolved, and 'influential allies' were available. The volatile pattern of political opportunities also provided 'unstable alignments' (Tarrow, 1998: 8589) as the state's own legislative framework on waste issues remained concentrated on profitability rather than sustainability, and provided local successes for regional campaigns. Ultimately, the Irish state's aim of eight regional incinerators was first reduced to just three (in Dublin, Meath and Cork), and even these now seem unlikely to be developed (Leonard et al, 2009)

The emergence of the Green Party as a government coalition partner from 2007 to 2011 has had mixed results in relation to incineration, with disagreement about three of the originally proposed eight incinerators continuing. Their combination of framing approaches, combined with the utilisation of EU directives as the basis for legal challenges, represented some success for community groups opposed to the state's waste policy. Plans for incinerators in Dublin (Poolbeg), Meath (with planning permission announced in July 2008) and Cork are still part of state policy, and campaigners have continued to oppose their introduction. However, the economic downturn has made the development of regional incinerators unlikely. The Irish Greens have been criticised for their participation in the last coalition government, but they have continued to resist attempts to introduce incineration in Dublin, Cork and Meath.

The Irish waste case studies demonstrate the complexities surrounding the issue of state or corporate plans for dealing with an ongoing waste management crisis in the face of local community concerns about the environment (see also Leonard, 2011). This chapter has demonstrated that from a governance perspective, the dichotomies that exist between centralised forms of power and community based movements derived from local political alliances indicates the need for local consultation at the planning and implementation level. While this may delay the introduction of critical infrastructure required by existing levels of consumption, the benefits for the wider political process would include an increased sense of confidence in the processes of development in regions that, for whatever reason, may feel marginalised from the central planning process. The responses of community groups in both jurisdictions can also be seen to have had an impact on local politics, and have provided an outlet for concerns about wider issues such as democratic deficit

The prevalence of community responses indicates the extent to which degrees of 'ecopopulist' (Szasz, 1994) local governmentality are manifested in Ireland's body politic across the island. Ultimately, this embedded form of community politics creates an initial but significant layer of civil society which provides an outlet for local political concerns about corporate or state activity, empowers local actors, instigates local political careers and augments local flows of knowledge and networking on issues such as health, politics and regional planning, thereby enhancing the political opportunity framework in a manner which goes beyond NIMBY concerns with the development of regional repertories of power. While such power is by its very nature transient and fleeting, the temporary leverage it provides creates moments of access for community activists in a manner that is rarely replicated. One recommendation that can emerge from this analysis is the necessity for policy makers to come to an understanding of community concerns about waste management and environmental issues, an. One way this can be achieved is through community mediation and forums, which allow for an expression of local narratives and sentiments. Ultimately, such local narratives can be seen to contribute to a broader understanding about what it is 'ecological modernisation' represents for a society where issues such as waste management and regional politics has a global resonance.

References

Blowers, A. (1987) 'Transition of transformation? Environmental policy under Thatcher', *Public Administration*, vol 65, p: 277–94.

Council of the European Communities (1991) *Council Directive 91/156/EEC of 18 March 1991 amending Directive 75/442/EEC on waste,* Brussels: Council of the European Communities

Council of the European Communities (1999) *Council Directive 1999/31/EC of 26 April 1999 on the landfill of waste*, Brussels: Council of the European Communities.

Department of the Environment (1994) *Recycling for Ireland*, Dublin: Government Publications.

Department of the Environment (1997) *Sustainable development: A strategy for Ireland* (April 1997) Dublin: Government Publications, www.environ.ie/en/Environment/LocalAgenda21/PublicationsDocuments/FileDownLoad,1825,en.pdf

Environmental Protection Agency (2000) *Ireland's environment: A millennium report*, Wexford: Environmental Protection Agency.

Environmental Protection Agency (2003) *The national waste interim report 2003*, Wexford: Environmental Protection Agency.

Environmental Protection Agency (2006) *National waste report: 2005 data update*, Wexford: Environmental Protection Agency

European Environment Agency (2002) *Europe's environment: The Second Assessment: State of the environment report no 2*, www.eea.europa.eu/publications/92-828-3351-8

Fingal County Council (2002) 'Minutes of meeting of county council', 5 March; www.fingalcoco.ie/minutes/meeting_fulldoc.aspx?id=488

Galway City Council (2001) *The Connacht waste plan*, Galway: City Council Office.

Government of Ireland (1998) *Changing our ways*, Policy Statement, Dublin: Department of Environment and Local Government.

Grove-White, R. (1993) 'Environmentalism: a new moral discourse for technological society', in Kay Milton (ed), *Environmentalism: The view from Anthropology*, London: Routledge.

Leonard, L. (2005) *Politics inflamed: GSE and the campaign against incineration in Ireland*, Ecopolitics series vol 1, Galway: Greenhouse Press/Choice Publishing.

Leonard, L. (2006) *Green nation: The Irish environmental movement from Carnsore Point to the Rossport 5*, Ecopolitics series vol 2, Galway: Greenhouse Press/Choice Publishing.

Leonard, L. (2008) *The environmental movement in Ireland*, Dordrecht: Springer.

Leonard, L. (2011) *Community campaigns for sustainable living: Health, waste and protest in civil society*, Advances in Ecopolitics vol 7, Bingley: Emerald.

Leonard, L., Doran, P. and Fagan, H. (2009) 'A burning issue? Governance and anti-incinerator campaigns in Ireland, North and South', *Environmental Politics*, vol 18, no 6, pp 896-91.

Rawcliffe, P. (1998) *Environmental pressure groups in transition*, Manchester: Manchester University Press.

Roberts, J. (2004) *Environmental policy*, London: Routledge

Rootes, C. and Leonard, L. (eds) (2010) *Environmental movements and waste infrastructure*, London: Taylor & Francis.

Szasz, A., (1994) *Eco-populism: Toxic waste and the movement for environmental justice*, London: UCL Press.

Tarrow, S. (1998) *Power in movement: Social movements and contentious politics* (2nd edn), Cambridge: Cambridge University Press.

Weale, A. (1992) *The new politics of pollution*, Manchester: Manchester University Press.

ELEVEN

Waste collection as an environmental justice issue: a case study of a neighbourhood in Bristol, UK

Karen Bell and David Sweeting

Introduction

Despite recent attempts to improve urban waste management through increased recycling, insufficient attention has been paid to the social and distributional impacts of waste policy. This omission means that such changes appear to have reinforced environmental injustices through the re/production of inequitable social burdens and benefits. This chapter argues that, if policy makers were to consider waste management through the frame of 'environmental justice', such problems could be avoided. This assertion is illustrated by analysing household waste and recycling in a disadvantaged neighbourhood in the city of Bristol, UK, where we are both resident. We provide evidence of unequal and unjust burdens faced by deprived communities in relation to waste collection services. Our aims are threefold. First, we intend to make an original contribution to the literature on environmental justice that, we consider, has overlooked the distributional aspects of municipal waste collection. Second, we aim to highlight the nature of the injustices that less well-off communities face in this regard, especially when compared to more resourceful actors who produce waste and profit from its sale. Third, we suggest ways that policy makers might ameliorate the injustices that occur in the processes of waste collection and recycling.

In this chapter we aim to make a contribution to the literature on waste from the discipline of social policy, a field of study that has been slow to catch on to the environmental debate (Fitzpatrick, 2011), despite the obvious links between the environment and poverty, disadvantage and inequality. We highlight the inadequacy of policy in this area, and demonstrate that, while there has been a welcome reduction in the amount of waste landfilled as a result of new waste collection policies, this has come at a cost to some of the households least able to bear it.

Although environmental justice is not inherently an urban issue – rural communities can also be affected – environmental justice discourse often has an urban focus. This is possibly because there are particular aspects of the unequal distribution of environmental goods and bads that are likely to be exacerbated, or have been shown to be more prominent, in the urban context, particularly in relation to urban air quality, access to green space, flood risk and the location of waste facilities (Walker, 2012). We consider that the issues raised in this chapter are likely to be illustrative of the sorts of concerns faced by less well-off urban communities in the global North where, in the face of increased waste production, alongside pressure to reduce the amount that goes to landfill, municipal authorities are reorganising their waste collection and disposal arrangements.

The next section outlines the idea of environmental justice and gives examples of how the concept has been linked to waste. Then, after describing the arrangements for the collection and disposal of household waste within the broader context of waste policy in the UK, this is related to environmental injustice. Using data gathered from householders in the case study neighbourhood, the analysis explores their views and experiences with regard to waste collection services. We conclude with reflections on the significance of this analysis for municipal waste policy.

Concept of environmental justice

As Walker (2012: 1) remarks, the term 'environmental justice' can be used as 'a campaigning slogan, as a description for academic research, as a policy principle, as an agenda and as a name given to a political movement'. These different uses reflect the growing awareness and importance of the concept in political, academic and policy contexts. In this chapter we consider 'environmental justice' in a broad sense, referring to the ideal of a healthy and safe environment for all, and a fair share of natural resources, access to environmental information and participation in environmental decision making. This conception is something of an extension of how the term was originally used. Most accounts pinpoint its emergence in the US from research (that is, Chavis and Lee, 1987) and protest, highlighting the location of toxic waste facilities in predominantly black and other minority ethnic neighbourhoods. Many subsequent studies demonstrated that poor and minority ethnic communities were more likely to live near to environmentally hazardous facilities and to receive little or inadequate legal protection (Bryant and Mohai, 1992; Lavelle and Coyle, 1992; Adeola, 1994; Cutter, 1995; Kratch, 1995). Thus, the term 'environmental justice' originally referred to the unequal sociospatial distribution of pollution, and a lack of redress for impacted groups. Moreover, the term and movement was initially bound up with considerations of waste.

However, the concept has travelled, expanded, and has been taken up by social movements, and, in some cases, by policy makers and environmental planners worldwide. Walker (2012) notes examples of the term now being used throughout Europe, as well as in Africa, South America, Australia and Taiwan. In the process of its dispersal and transfer, the term 'environmental justice' has been interpreted in different ways and has become more contested and contentious. It has now been applied with regard to environmental disparities or injustice, not only on the grounds of 'race', but also class, disability, gender and nation (see, for example, Buckingham-Hatfield et al, 2005). It now includes normative demands and expectations across a number of different policy domains (Stephens et al, 2001; Lucas et al, 2004), spreading to encompass broadly drawn environmental considerations, taking in matters such as air quality, water contamination, flooding, noise, transport and fuel poverty, to name only a few (Walker, 2012).

While many analysts focus on particular dimensions of the term, we argue that environmental justice should be seen as encompassing all of the following aspects, so that the potential for resolution in one dimension will not create a problem in another:

- Distributive justice, concerned with how environmental 'goods' (for example, access to green space) and environmental 'bads' (for example, pollution) are distributed among different groups.
- Procedural justice, encompassing access to information and the fairness or equity of access to environmental decision-making processes.
- Recognition justice, pertaining to the need to respect, include and value oppressed groups.
- Substantive justice, considering the quality of the environment.
- Policy justice, concerned with the outcomes of environmental policy decisions and how these have an impact on different social groups.
- Intranational justice, which focuses on how these distributions and processes occur within a country.
- International justice, which includes international and global disparities and processes.

- Intergenerational justice, which is concerned with fairness and responsibility towards future generations.

For more discussion on these dimensions of environmental justice, see Bell (2013: forthcoming). Although the focus in this chapter is on on distributive, procedural and policy justice in this discussion, the argument also takes into account the other aspects listed above.

In the UK, there is still only limited awareness of environmental justice in most academic and policy contexts, despite an outbreak of interest between the mid-1990s and the 2000s. One of the key studies during this period was that of the UK Sustainable Development Research Network (SDRN) whose evidence review concluded that 'environmental injustice is a real and substantive problem within the UK' (Lucas et al, 2004: 2). This was based on an appraisal of a number of UK studies showing sociospatial environmental disparities based on income, that is, that deprived areas were more likely to experience higher levels of pollution, fuel poverty, transportation inequities and lack of access to healthy food and green space than their better-off counterparts (DoE, 1996; DETR, 1998, 2001; Boardman et al, 1999; Donkin et al, 1999; FoE, 1999; McLaren et al, 1999; Agyeman, 2000; ESRC, 2001; Lucas et al, 2004). Other studies showed that that disadvantaged communities rarely had influence over environmental decision making (Evans and Percy, 1999; Brown, 2000), thereby experiencing procedural and recognition injustice. Following these findings, the Blair and Brown Labour governments made a number of comments that indicated recognition of the problem of environmental injustice, although they generally shied away from using the term, referring instead to 'environmental inequality', or 'environment and social justice' (Eames, 2006).

Waste and environmental justice

Most studies on environmental justice and waste have concentrated on the location of waste facilities – such as landfill sites and incinerators – and their impacts on health, pollution and noise in the neighbourhoods where such facilities are located. Both landfill sites and incinerators have been associated with some reproductive and cancer outcomes, although there have been some mixed results as a result of methodological complexities (Vrijheid, 2000; Rushton, 2003; Franchini et al, 2004; Petts, 2005; Saunders, 2007; Porta et al, 2009).

The relationship between landfill sites is similarly complex in relation to patterns of social deprivation. For example, a study of 21 hazardous waste sites in five European countries concluded that there was no overall evidence that more deprived communities lived near to landfill sites (Dolk et al, 1998). In England, Elliott et al (2001) found that 80 per cent of the population lived within two kilometres of some kind of landfill site. However, the Environment Agency's study of landfill sites in England found that a greater proportion of landfill sites were in the more deprived wards (Environment Agency, 2002). Wheeler (2004), examining landfill sites for England and Wales, found that the relationship between a 'landfill index' and deprivation varied between urban and rural wards. He noted that there were 'complex associations' so that, in totally urban wards, a weak trend towards landfill sites being found in less deprived wards was observed, whereas this was not the case in rural or semi-urban areas. However, the most recent review of the literature on waste management covering Europe and the US found 'consistent indications' that waste facilities were often disproportionally located in areas with more deprived residents, adding 'This applies to waste incinerators, landfills, hazardous waste sites, legal and illegal' (Martuzzi et al, 2010: 21). Thus the evidence for landfill sites is mixed.

The point of departure from these studies is that there are other environmental justice considerations at play in the operation of waste services. This chapter concentrates on how municipal waste policies concerning the collection of waste from households in the case study neighbourhood contribute to environmental injustice. This theme links to other research on the quality of services in neighbourhoods. Evidence from national surveys of poverty and social exclusion shows that local environmental services are particularly likely to be inadequate in deprived areas (Bramley and Fisher, 2006). In addition, Hastings et al (2005) identify the structural factors that create a more challenging context for waste and other cleansing service provision in poorer neighbourhoods. They note that there may be more need for waste collection in deprived areas because often more people live in each household, because there is a greater use of cheaper and more heavily packaged food, because household items may be of inferior quality and, therefore, not last as long and because poorer people are less likely to have a car with which to dispose of items themselves. Their study implies that achieving good outcomes within neighbourhoods depends on service provision being appropriate to the local context. Further work suggests that if good outcomes are to be achieved in all neighbourhoods, then there may be a need to reconfigure or redistribute service provision (Hastings, 2007).

Public services are now also being required to be more responsive to consumers. Some consumers are more influential than others and evidence suggests that certain groups have a stronger voice, for example, older, educated, middle-class groups. Consequently, they are more likely to be able to influence service delivery to favour their own area (Hastings, 2009). This process may be exacerbated in the contemporary political and economic climate as waste collection services are potential targets for contracting out, driving down pay and working conditions. This can risk quality, especially in less vociferous areas.

UK municipal waste policy

Municipal waste policy in the UK is driven at a national level by the Department for Environment, Food and Rural Affairs (DEFRA) and, to a lesser extent, by the Department for Trade and Industry (DTI) and the Department for Communities and Local Government (CLG). Key legislation in this field includes the Environmental Protection Act 1990 and the Waste Minimisation Act 1998. In common with other European countries, national waste policy also operates within the remit of the EU landfill directive, requiring year-on-year reductions in the amount of waste sent to landfill (Bulkeley et al, 2005). Consequently, much individual municipality policy – such as that of Bristol City Council – in the area of household waste is constrained and prompted by national and international policy.

Therefore, expectations placed on local authorities in waste and recycling have increased markedly. Until recently, little more was required of local authorities than to arrange the collection of waste from households, and to organise its disposal into landfill (Bulkeley et al, 2005). However, since the passing of the EU landfill directive, and its conversion into UK waste policy in the waste strategy 2000 (DETR, 2000), local authorities have been required to hit increasingly demanding targets on the reduction of waste. Restrictions on the ability of local authorities to use landfill has led to them exploring options around the reduction of waste, increased recycling and alternatives to landfill for non-recyclable residual waste.

However, such a move away from landfill has been a difficult and contested process, with alternative waste treatment options such as anaerobic digestion and mechanical biological treatment either seen as undesirable or too expensive (Entwistle et al, 2007). It has also required much greater collaboration between local authorities in order to cope with more demanding waste treatment arrangements. Previously, collaboration was necessary between district councils as waste collection authorities, and county councils as waste disposal authorities. However, now many more authorities are collaborating much more closely in sub-regional partnerships in order to take advantage of economies of scale to process waste and recycling appropriately (Entwistle et al, 2007), something that was previously unnecessary.

In national waste policy documents there is little recognition of the concept of environmental justice, either explicitly or implicitly. For example, DEFRA (2011) gives much consideration to the economic and environmental impacts of waste and waste policy, but much less to its social impacts. There is concern with avoiding placing burdens on business, and on reflecting the needs of different sorts of businesses, but much less on avoiding burdens on households. Communities are primarily presented as consumers and producers of waste, although there is some mention of the importance of civil society in dealing with waste (DEFRA, 2011: 52). Where social impacts are discussed, this tends to be in terms of the 'irresponsible minority' (2011: 45) who engage in fly-tipping and other anti-social littering or disposal. There is no consideration that residents may be ordinary, responsible citizens who might, for various reasons, find it difficult to meet the obligations imposed on them by policies designed to cut the amount sent to landfill by increasing recycling. There is little treatment of people in any socially differentiated way. Emphasis on having waste arrangements to suit local circumstances tends to be couched in terms of facilitating greater citizen involvement as part of the 'Big Society' in recycling, rather than recognition of the genuine difficulties that disadvantaged people may face in complying with waste arrangements. Indeed, Section 46 of the Environmental Protection Act 1990 enables local authorities to impose penalties on householders who present their waste incorrectly for collection.

This pressure on households, rather than business, is a result of a policy framework that favours recycling, rather than reduction, of waste. There have been attempts to persuade producers to reduce packaging (see, for example, DEFRA, 2006), and specific EU legislation introduced in the UK in 1997 (The Packaging and Packaging Waste Directive 94/62/EC) that requires packaging to be minimised and to be designed for recovery and reuse. However, it seems that implementation of the Waste Directive has largely focused on recovery rather than reduction (INCPEN, 2012; Valpak, 2012). In addition, small companies are exempt, and there are a number of private companies that run 'exemption schemes' (for example, Valpak).

As mentioned previously, considerable progress in the UK has been made in moving household waste away from landfill towards different forms of recycling (DEFRA, 2011). However, while diverting waste from landfill has been relatively successful, waste prevention has not, according to Wrap, the government's waste adviser (Wrap, 2011). Targets do not appear to have been met with regard to reduction of waste production. At the time of writing, retailers have not yet met Phase 2 of the voluntary Courtauld Commitment, which pledged to reduce product and packaging waste in the grocery supply chain by 5 per cent – having reduced it by only 0.4 per cent since the pledge was made in 2010 (Wrap, 2011).

It is estimated that one quarter to one third of domestic waste is made up of packaging (The Open University, 2008; City of York Council, 2012), yet businesses appear, on the whole, unwilling to reduce their packaging. This may be a result of commercial interests. As one non-governmental organisation (NGO) describes, 'the problem is that packaging is driven by the desire to promote brands and make money' (Green Choices, 2012: 1). Thus, householders are carrying the burden of disposing of packaging produced to increase business sales. This is a clear injustice, with commercial interests benefiting at the cost of householders.

Waste and environmental justice in a disadvantaged area of Bristol, UK

The case study focused on Lockleaze, an outer city estate in Bristol with multiple indicators of deprivation (ODPM, 2004), including income deprivation, employment deprivation, health deprivation and disability, education, skills and training deprivation, barriers to housing and services, living environment and crime. Part of the ward is one of the 10 per cent most deprived areas of England (Bristol City Council, 2008). There is a high concentration of disadvantaged groups, such as older people, minority ethnic people, people with disabilities and people living on low incomes (Bristol City Council, 2008). A large proportion of residents (34 per cent) live in houses rented from the City Council (ONS, 2001). Particular problems in the area are unemployment, high levels of road accidents, poor health, low levels of educational attainment and lack of facilities (ONS, 2001; Bristol City Council, 2008). Life expectancy is two years less than the Bristol average, and six years less than the wealthiest wards in Bristol (DoH, 2006). There are few shops in the area and little provision of fresh, healthy food (Lockleaze Neighbourhood Trust, 2006). Most people have to go out of the area to shop, yet 32 per cent of the people have no car or van (ONS, 2001). In general, there are few amenities in the area and, since 2000, Lockleaze has lost a number of facilities including the local Area Housing Office, the secondary school, a primary school and a local resource centre. The area does have more than the average amount of green space for Bristol (Bristol City Council, 2011), but most of this space has no trees, landscaping, play facilities, seating or any other facilities.

In line with national policy, Bristol's waste management has focused on recycling, as opposed to reduction, of waste. It has been very successful in terms of recycling, with recycling rates reported to have risen from 12.8 per cent in 2004/05, to 37.3 per cent in 2008/09, and the rate expected to rise to 46 per cent in 2011/12 (*Bristol Evening Post*, 2011; *The Guardian*, 2011). The arrangements for the collection of household waste from most households in Bristol at the time of the research, and now, was/is as follows: fortnightly 'kerbside' collections of waste destined for landfill in the form of either one 'wheelie bin' or four waste sacks; weekly collections of recyclable material – cardboard, paper, glass and many other items mixed in one black box; and weekly collections of food waste in a brown bin.

These services are free at the point of use, although other waste collections incur charges so that large items (for example, mattresses or fridges) are collected on an agreed date for a charge of £15 for a collection of up to three items. A garden waste bin is also available to householders for an annual charge of £32 (reduced to £29 should householders pay by direct debit), plus an initial charge of £21 for the supply of the bin. Residents on some Council Tax or Housing Benefits can claim a 50 per cent discount. This is still a substantial cost to benefit claimants as, for example, current benefit income for a single person, excluding rent, is £67.50. Residents also pay a local 'council tax' (a property tax) which all households are obliged to pay, unless they are students or in receipt of benefits. Local authority spending is largely paid for out of the Council Tax, grants from central government and taxes on businesses.

Fifteen Lockleaze residents were interviewed between July and August 2007, all members of the Lockleaze Environment Group (LEG). A further focus group of six LEG members was carried out in August 2011. The sample was selected through 'convenience sampling' (Robson, 2002), using people who were willing to be interviewed. One of the authors of this chapter (Karen Bell) is a member of LEG and the other (David Sweeting) is a local resident. Because of our 'insider' status, it was not considered possible to be 'value free', but rather we aimed to be 'reflexive', that is, aware of our subjective position at all times while attempting to see beyond it.

The interviews and focus group findings illustrate policy injustice with regard to some waste services. For example, in the area of 'green waste', green or garden waste had previously been routinely collected as part of normal collection procedures. Now, however, residents are no longer allowed to dispose of waste in the landfill container. This is positive in terms of substantive environmental justice, as green waste produces methane gas, but, in Bristol, residents have to pay for its removal and recycling, as described earlier. This creates difficulties for some residents, who find they are unable to pay the charge:

> 'The green stuff from the garden, garden waste, they don't come and collect it. You have to pay and I can't afford it so the green stuff, there is so much of it, with all the branches, I can't take it to the tip.... So that is a problem – it all piles up in my garden and takes up space where I want to grow food.' (participant 1, Lockleaze Environment Group Focus Group [LEGFG])

The lack of free green waste collection creates difficulties, not only for the poorer residents themselves, but also for the entire community, as people attempt to dispose of this waste in the most economical manner. Therefore, some residents responded to the build-up of green waste by burning it in their gardens:

> 'On a Sunday night it's like Beirut with all the garden waste being burnt so it is a big issue, you know, how to get rid of it.' (participant 6, LEGFG)

Such fires clearly constitute a fire risk, and cause local air pollution. Additionally, such fires can cause friction between members of the community:

> 'There's fires all through the summer ... one day they had to get the fire brigade out. People are burning the waste because they can't afford to get it collected.... If you ring up and complain about the fires they want to know the address but then the neighbour gets in trouble, maybe a fine ... that does not solve the problem because nearly everyone is doing it.' (participant 5, LEGFG)

Similar problems were also caused by payment for the collection and disposal of large household items (for example, furniture). Residents without either access to a car to enable them to take large items to the municipal dump, or the means to pay for the collection of large items, are disadvantaged:

> 'I've got things that I need to get taken to the tip but I've got no way of getting them to the tip because I haven't got a car ... so it ends up hanging around the house.... When I peg out [that is, die] someone's gonna have a horrible job cleaning out my rubbish ... things that don't work anymore, stuff like that.' (participant 3, LEGFG)

> 'If we had something, even a van that came round. Years ago, if you had a big item, you could ring the Council and they would come and get it. But now they charge you. I had a sofa and I wanted to give it to the Sofa Project [a voluntary organisation that gives unwanted furniture to people on low incomes] but you have to take it to them and we didn't have the transport. Now we've got to pay for the Council to take it.' (participant 2, LEGFG)

Another resident commented:

> 'A neighbour has the whole shed full of stuff that needs to go in a skip but she can't afford it and she can't afford to get it collected ... and she keeps putting more in there ... it's not healthy.' (participant 5, LEGFG)

There are also increasing controls on where people can take their waste, so that residents can no longer use the nearest site in a neighbouring local authority area:

> 'I heard they were going to have "meet and greet people" at the waste sites in South Gloucestershire. I thought that was a good idea and then I realised it is just so people from Bristol can't use it. So if you live on the border, like we do, you would not then be able to go to the nearest one. That seems ludicrous ... I thought it sounded so nice but then I realised that. That means we have to go further ... we can't just take it to the nearest place ... you will have to produce ID.' (participant 2, LEGFG)

Some of the residents also said they had difficulty coping with the infrequency of the fortnightly collection, or knew people who did, particularly some people with disabilities, older people or people with young families who may need to dispose of sanitary waste:

> 'Flies, maggots, smell! It's disgusting. Since they brought the recycling in [implemented the policy] the rubbish bin only gets emptied once a fortnight now. It's disgusting. It's a health hazard. I've never seen so many rats round here in my life. My cats bring back at least seven or eight a week.... Before they never brought back any.' (respondent B, Interview)

Residents did not just blame the local authority for the waste problems, however; they also pointed to the underlying issues that created waste problems in the first place, such as the short lifetime of the goods they purchased. One resident said:

> 'Things now break down much quicker.... When it's just outside the warranty, usually, that's when it breaks down [laughs] ... so you have to keep buying more....' (participant 2, LEGFG)

As mentioned previously, studies show that waste is more of an issue for poor people as they have to replace their items more often as they are less able to afford durable, high-quality items (see, for example, Hastings et al, 2005; Hastings, 2007). Those on low incomes are also less able to get their items repaired, as it is cheaper to replace them. Moreover, recent studies show that a number of income-deprived groups also tend to experience 'time poverty' as a result of, for example, caring responsibilities, or long hours of work (Burchardt, 2008). These groups include people with young families, single parents, carers and those on low wages who have to work excessive hours. Putting the emphasis on household recycling instead of reducing waste at source tends to be more of a burden for low-income families because of the time it takes up. The respondents alluded to a shortage of time on a number of occasions. One resident asserted:

> 'It's putting everything on the individual. I mean, why should we be messing around with waste? The Council don't have to do so much now as we have to spend time sorting it and its like with the electric, before they used to come and read the meters, they employed people to do that. Now they've laid them all off and we have to do it ourselves.' (participant 6, LEGFG)

Thus, there was some recognition that the time burden of waste management was falling on the community. Moreover, there was considerable evidence that residents felt poorly treated in their dealings with the Council and in the level of their engagement with decision-making processes, indicating not only distributional injustice, but also procedural and recognition injustice. There was articulation of a broader discontent with the Council in relation to environmental matters in Lockleaze. Such sentiments echo many studies of public participation (see, for example, Dargan, 2004), with residents disappointed with the level, form and extent of response offered to them by public authorities. In the earlier stage of the research, residents commented:

> 'Central government tell the Council what to do so, even if they do hear what you say, they then go away and make a different decision. They don't take your view into account but they can tick the box to say that they have consulted.' (respondent K, interview)

> 'They seem to walk all over us or send us people who don't care who aren't from the area. They go back and say what we want and then it just gets chucked in the bin.' (respondent J, interview)

Other respondents commented on the apparently unequal power relations between residents and the community on one side, and on governmental authorities on the other, caused by differences in position, access to information, and control of process:

> '... it seems that those who manage the community, they don't live here so they don't know what the real problems we face and what really make us happy. They do what is good for them. Whatever the agenda is I think it is purely politics. They had a specific agenda and when we are asking for some of the things that might disturb their programme or agenda ... they don't go along with our request.' (respondent F, interview)

> 'It's difficult to find out what's going on.... If it wasn't for the Lockleaze Environment Group I wouldn't find out anything because the Council don't send out leaflets or anything telling you what they are doing.' (respondent G, interview)

Others seemed to tire of the effort involved with attempting to involve and inform themselves of local processes:

> 'There's a lot of muddying the waters that goes on so you can't really follow what's happening. They don't follow the processes they are supposed to or reply to things. You just end up getting confused and give up.' (respondent P, interview)

> 'I've noticed a distinct increase in bullying, instead of calm discussion [in the Council meetings]. You end up feeling hurt and disgusted and demoralised.' (respondent D, interview)

After these interviews, many of these residents were engaged in a community planning process to produce a 'Lockleaze Vision'. This was also a frustrating process for many of them as they described on their website:

> Overall, the document presents a very negative picture of Lockleaze ... in order to justify the drastic changes the council wants to make ie, to use Lockleaze to raise money by selling off the land for property development.... Members of Lockleaze Environment Group do not want any of this and we attended the meetings of Lockleaze Voice for over three years to put forward these points, but our ideas were not allowed to go in the main part of the document (they were placed separately at the back). Most LEG members dropped out of the process with frustration. (LEG, 2011)

As Burton (2003) notes, many analysts blame deprived communities themselves for their lack of influence on local decision-making processes, alleging that they are uninterested and apathetic. This is supported by the post-material values thesis (Inglehart, 1990), which suggests that poorer people are too preoccupied with meeting their basic needs for food, warmth and security to be able to think about, or be active on, environmental issues. However, there is now a growing body of evidence that is challenging this view, suggesting that the affect of demographic factors on environmental attitudes has been exaggerated and misrepresented (Buttel, 1987; Jones and Dunlap, 1992). Some of these studies have tended to base their conclusions on purchasing decisions or 'green consumerism', which clearly limits the perceived 'environmentalism' of the poor, since environmentally friendly products tend to be more expensive and less available in deprived areas. In general, there is evidence of high levels of sustained community activity in disadvantaged areas (Dinham, 2005). However, people in deprived communities need to see results in order to sustain motivation (Burningham and Thrush, 2001; Brown, 2002), and want to work on their own agendas rather than those imposed on them (CDP, 1977).

As members of the local environment group, all the participants in the case study were committed environmentalists, but as people on low incomes, they were unable to comply with the waste management systems. As one participant pointed out, the burden of waste management was falling on the community – the council had not taken any initiative to reduce the source of the waste, for example, by creating by-laws to so that manufacturers would have to reduce their packaging.

Conclusion

The first conclusion that we can draw from this analysis is that there is clear evidence of environmental injustice in relation to waste in the case study neighbourhood. This is illustrated most starkly as policy injustice, as it arose out of the impacts of policies in place that were, ironically, ultimately designed to reduce environmental degradation. It appears that some of these policies were clearly counter-productive (for example, causing some income-deprived residents to light fires in order to dispose of waste). Others might not have been environmentally counter-productive, in the sense that they were still effective in diverting waste from landfill, but are surely unjust in the sense that they have had a disproportionate impact on those with least income.

Second, we also point to the lack of recognition of the issue of environmental justice in policies designed to reduce waste. This was evident, not only when analysing the text of relevant policy documents, but also in the attitudes of public authorities as perceived by residents, providing clear evidence of a lack of recognition of justice and procedural justice. In 2005, the Labour government ratified the United Nations Economic Commission for Europe (UNECE) Aarhus Convention, which grants the public rights regarding access to information, public participation and access to justice, in governmental decision-making processes on matters concerning the local, national and transboundary environment (UNECE, 1999). However, it appears that the local council were not implementing this Convention in the area.

Third, and most importantly, by focusing on community recycling rather than reducing waste, especially packaging, the burden of waste management has fallen on householders rather than the companies that produce the waste. These companies benefit from the advertising carried on their packaging, as well as the extra sales resulting from the continual need to replace their short-life products. Thus, they profit from waste management policies that focus largely on recycling rather than the three steps that should come before that – reducing, reusing and repairing. Unless these three steps are prioritised, unnecessary waste will still have to be managed, burdening the taxpayer, the householder, future generations, and possibly people in low-income countries whose governments may agree to import waste from other countries.

It appears that it is national, rather than local, processes that are driving these problems. Progress on environmental justice may have been seriously undermined by the Coalition government's decision to abolish the Sustainable Development Commission in 2011, whose role it was to hold the government to account over environmental matters, and who were actively progressing the environmental justice agenda. However, local government does have the power to implement some changes so as to alleviate this injustice. This analysis suggests a number of measures would be helpful both in reducing waste and in reducing environmental justice in waste policy. We recommend the following minimum changes to local authority policies and procedures:

- implement the Aarhus Convention;
- carry out equalities impact assessments on waste management processes;
- advise consumers that they can report over-packaging to the local Trading Standards Department (for example, see City of York Council, 2012);
- create by-laws with strict standards that will force companies to reduce their packaging;
- make all waste collection – whether destined for landfill or for recycling – free at the point of use;
- encourage and offer incentives for companies to produce reusable, compostable and recyclable packaging as part of a wider effort to eliminate unnecessary packaging.

Waste collection services are an environmental justice issue, creating uneven benefits and burdens and deepening social disparities. There is much that local authorities and other policy makers could do to turn this situation around, but ultimately, citizens should begin to demand that unnecessary waste is no longer produced.

References

Adeola, F. (1994) 'Environmental hazards, health, and racial inequity in hazardous waste distribution', *Environment and Behavior*, vol 26, pp 99-126.

Agyeman, J. (2000) *Environmental justice: From the margins to the mainstream*, London: Town and Country Planning Association.

Bell, K. (2013: forthcoming) *Environmental justice: Political, economic and cultural foundations*, Bristol: The Policy Press.

Boardman, B., Bullock, S. and McLaren, D, (1999) *Equity and the environment: Guidelines for green and socially just government*, London: Catalyst Trust and Friends of the Earth.

Bramley, G. and Fisher, T. (2006) 'Poverty and local services', in C. Pantazis, D. Gordon and R. Levitas (eds) *Poverty and social exclusion in Britain*, Bristol: The Policy Press.

Bristol City Council (2008) 'Bristol City Council ward profiles 2008 – Lockleaze' (www.bristol.gov.uk/WardFinder?XSL=warddetail&WardId=19).

Bristol City Council (2011) *Quality of life in Bristol* (www.bristol.gov.uk/node/4103).

Bristol Evening Post (2011) 'Bristol City Council bags up leaves in plastic for burial in landfill' (www.thisisbristol.co.uk/Bristol-City-Council-bags-leaves-plastic-burial/story-14018529-detail/story.html).

Brown, A.P. (2000) 'Environmental justice: Views from the Black environmental network environmental justice seminar', Friends of the Earth/London School of Hygiene and Tropical Medicine at WHO Ministers Conference on Environment and Health, June 1999, London.

Brown, A.P. (2002) *Community involvement: Findings from working for communities*, Development Department Research Programme Research Findings no 137, Edinburgh: Scottish Executive Research Unit.

Bryant, B. and Mohai, P. (eds) (1992) *Race and the incidence of environmental hazards: A time for discourse*, Boulder, CO: Westview Press.

Buckingham-Hatfield, S., Reeves, D. and Batchelor A. (2005) 'Wasting women: The environmental justice of including women in municipal waste management', *Local Environment*, vol 10, pp 427-44.

Bulkeley, H., Askins, K., Watson, M., Hudson, R. and Weaver, P. (2005) *Governing waste sustainably – Challenges and opportunities*, Durham: Durham University.

Burchardt, T. (2008) *Time and income poverty*, London: Centre for Analysis of Social Exclusion, London School of Economics (http://sticerd.lse.ac.uk/dps/case/cr/CASEreport57.pdf).

Burningham, K. and Thrush, D. (2001) *Rainforests are a long way from here: The environmental concerns of disadvantaged groups*, York: Joseph Rowntree Foundation.

Burton, P. (2003) *Community involvement in neighbourhood regeneration: Stairway to heaven or road to nowhere?*, CNR Paper 13 (www.bristol.ac.uk/sps/cnrpaperspdf/cnr13sum.pdf).

Buttel, F.H. (1987) 'New directions in environmental sociology', *Annual Review of Sociology*, vol 13, pp 465-88.

CDP (Community Development Projects) (1977) *Gilding the ghetto: The state and the poverty experiments*, London: CDP.

Chavis, B.F. Jr., and Lee, C. (1987) *Toxic wastes and race in the United States*, New York: United Church of Christ Commission for Racial Justice.

City of York Council (2012) (www.york.gov.uk/info/200349/reduce_reuse_and_recycle/766/packaging_waste).

Cutter, S. (1995) 'Race, class and environmental justice', *Progress in Human Geography*, vol 19, pp 107-18.

Dargan, L. (2004) *A new approach to regeneration? Reflections on the New Deal for communities in Newcastle Upon Tyne*, Newcastle: Centre for Urban and Regional Development Studies, University of Newcastle upon Tyne.

DEFRA (Department for Environment, Food and Rural Affairs) (2006) *Saving money by reducing waste: Waste minimisation manual: A practical guide for farmers and growers* (www.defra.gov.uk/publications/files/pb11674-waste-minimisation-060508.pdf).

DEFRA (2011) *Government review of waste policy in England* (www.defra.gov.uk/publications/2011/06/14/pb13540-waste-review).

DETR (Department of the Environment, Transport and the Regions) (1998) *The impact of large foodstores on market towns and district centres*, London: The Stationery Office.

DETR (2000) *Waste strategy 2000*, London: The Stationery Office.

DETR (2001) *Road accident involvement of children from ethnic minorities*, London: The Stationery Office.

Dinham, A. (2005) 'Empowered or over-powered? The real experiences of local participation in the UK's New Deal for Communities', *Community Development Journal*, vol 40, no 3, pp 301-12.

DoE (Department of the Environment) (1996) *English House Condition Survey*, London: DoE.

DoH (Department of Health) (2006) *Health profile for Bristol* (www.communityhealthprofiles.info/profiles/hp2006/lo_res/00HB-HP2006.pdf).

Dolk, H., Vrijheid, M., Armstrong, B., Abramsky, L., Bianchi, F., Game, F., Nelen, V., Robert, E., Scott, J.E.S., Stone, D. and Tenconi, R. (1998) 'Risk of congenital abnormalities near hazardous waste landfill sites in Europe: the EUROHAZCON study', *The Lancet*, vol 352, pp 423-7.

Donkin, A., Dowler, E., Stevenson, S. and Turner, S. (1999) 'Mapping access to food at a local level', *British Food Journal*, vol 101, no 7, pp 554-64, in K. Burningham and D. Thrush (2001) *Rainforests are a long way from here: The environmental concerns of disadvantaged groups*, York: Joseph Rowntree Foundation.

Eames, M. (2006) *Reconciling environmental and social concerns: Findings from the JRF research programme*, York: Joseph Rowntree Foundation.

Elliott, P., Briggs, D., Morris, S., de Hoogh, C., Hurt, C., Jensen, T.K., Maitland, I., Richardson, S., Wakefield, J. and Jarup, L. (2001) 'Risk of adverse birth outcomes in populations living near landfill sites', *British Medical Journal*, vol 323, pp 363-8.

Entwistle, T, with Darlow, A., Downe, J., Dowson, L., Gains, F., John, P., Greasley, S., Sweeting, D. and Turner, K. (2007) *Perspectives on place shaping and service delivery*, Cardiff: Centre for Local and Regional Government Research, Cardiff University.

Environment Agency (2002) *The urban environment in England and Wales: A detailed assessment*, Bristol: Environment Agency.

ESRC (Economic and Social Research Council) (2001) *Environmental justice: Rights and means to a healthy environment for all*, Special Briefing No 7, University of Sussex.

Evans, B. and Percy, S. (1999) 'The opportunities and challenges for local environmental policy and action in the UK', in S. Buckingham-Hatfield and S. Percy *Constructing local environmental agendas*, Abingdon: Psychology Press, pp 172-84.

Fitzpatrick, T. (2011) 'Introduction', in T. Fitzpatrick (ed) *Understanding the environment and social policy*, Bristol: The Policy Press, pp 1-16.

FoE (Friends of the Earth) (1999) *Pollution injustice and the geographic relation between household income and polluting factories*, London: FoE (www.foe.co.uk/resource/reports/income_pollution.html).

Franchini, M., Rial, M., Buiatti, E. and Bianchi, F. (2004) 'Health effects of exposure to waste incinerator emissions: a review of epidemiological studies', *Ann Ist Super Sanita*, vol 40, pp 101-15.

Green Choices (2012) 'Packaging', www.greenchoices.org/green-living/food-drink/packagin2).

Guardian, The (2011) 'England's recycling rate has increased: get the data for your area', 7 January (www.guardian.co.uk/news/datablog/2011/jan/07/household-waste-recycling-by-area).

Hastings, A. (2007) 'Territorial justice and neighbourhood environmental services: a comparison of provision to deprived and better off neighbourhoods in the UK', *Environment and Planning C: Government and Policy*, vol 25, no 6, pp 896-917.

Hastings, A. (2009) 'Poor neighbourhoods and poor services: evidence on the "rationing" of environmental service provision to deprived neighbourhoods', *Urban Studies*, vol 46, no 13, pp 2907-27.

Hastings, A., Flint, J., McKenzie, C. and Mills, C. (2005) *Cleaning up neighbourhoods: Environmental problems and service provision in deprived areas*, Bristol: The Policy Press.

INCPEN (Industrial Council for Packaging and the Environment) (2012) *Legislation: Packaging and the environment* (www.incpen.org/displayarticle.asp?a=11&c=2).

Inglehart, R. (1990) *Culture shift in advanced industrial society*, Princeton, NJ: Princeton University Press

Jones, R.E. and Dunlap, R.E. (1992) 'The social bases of environmental concern: have they changed over time?', *Rural Sociology*, vol 57, no 1, pp 28-47

Kratch, K. (1995) 'Special report on environmental justice: grassroots reach the Whitehouse lawn', *Environmental Solutions*, vol 8, no 5, pp 68-77.

Lavelle, M. and Coyle, M. (1992) 'Unequal protection: the racial divide in environmental law', *The National Law Journal*, pp S1-S2.

LEG (Lockleaze Environment Group) (2011) *What is wrong with the 'Lockleaze Vision' plan?* (http://lockleaze.wordpress.com/2011/05/09/what-is-wrong-with-the-%E2%80%98lockleaze-vision%E2%80%99-pla2).

Lockleaze Neighbourhood Trust (2006) *Lockleaze community market evaluation report*, Bristol: Lockleaze Neighbourhood Trust.

Lucas, K., Walker, G., Eames, M., Fay, H. and Poustie, M. (2004) *Environment and social justice: Rapid research and evidence review*, London: Policy Studies Institute.

Murray, R. (1999) *Creating wealth from waste*, London: Demos.

McLaren, D., Cottray, O., Taylor, M., Pipes, S. and Bullock, S. (1999) *Pollution injustice: The geographic relation between household income and polluting factories*, London: Friends of the Earth (www.foe.org.uk/pollutioninjustice/poll-inj.html).

Martuzzi, M., Mitis, F. and Forastiere, F. (2010) 'Inequalities, inequities, environmental justice in waste management and health', *European Journal of Public Health*, vol 20, no 1, pp 21-6

ODPM (Office of the Deputy Prime Minister) (2004) *The English Indices of Deprivation* (www.communities.gov.uk/pub/443/Indicesofdeprivation2004summaryrevisedPDF154Kb_id1128443.pd2).

ONS (Office for National Statistics) (2001) *Census data* (www.bristol.gov.uk/statistics and www.neighbourhood.statistics.gov.u2).

Open University, The (2008) *The Open University household waste study: Key findings for 2007*, London: Department for the Environment, Food and Rural Affairs.

Petts, J. (2005) 'Enhancing environmental equity through decision making: learning from waste management', *Local Environment*, vol 10, no 4, pp 1–13

Porta, D., Milani, S., Lazzarino, A.I., Perucci, C.A. and Forastiere, F. (2009) 'Systematic review of epidemiological studies on health effects associated with management of solid waste', *Environmental Health*, vol 8, no 60, pp 1-14.

Robson, C. (2002) *Real world research: A resource for social scientists and practitioner-researchers*, Oxford: Blackwell.

Rushton, L. (2003) 'Health hazards and waste management', *British Medical Bulletin*, vol 68, pp 183–97

Saunders, P. (2007) 'A systematic review of the evidence of an increased risk of adverse birth outcomes in populations living in the vicinity of landfill waste disposal sites', in F. Mitis and M. Martuzzi (eds) *Population health and waste management: Scientific data and policy options*, Report of a WHO workshop, Rome, Italy, 29-30 March. Copenhagen: Regional Office for Europe, pp 2-27, Geneva: World Health Organization.

Stephens, C., Bullock, S. and Scott, A. (2001) *Environmental justice rights and means to a healthy environment for all*, Special Briefing Paper, Economic and Social Research Council, Global Environmental Change Programme, Brighton: ESRC Global Environmental Change Programme, University of Sussex (www.foe.co.uk/resource/reports/environmental_justice.pdf).

UNECE (United Nations Economic Commission on the Environment) (1999) *Convention on access to information, public participation in decision making and access to justice in environmental matters*, Geneva: UNECE

Valpak (2012) 'About us' (www.valpak.co.uk/AboutUs/Company/CompanyHistory.aspx1).

Vrijheid, M. (2000) 'Health effects of residence near hazardous waste landfill sites: a review of epidemiologic literature', *Environmental Health Perspectives*, vol 108, suppl 1, pp 101-2E.

Walker, G. (2012) *Environmental justice: Concepts, evidence, and politics*, London: Routledе.

Wheeler, B.W. (2004) 'Health-related environmental indices and environmental equity in England and Wales', *Environment and Planning A*, vol 36, no 5, pp 803-22.

Wrap (2011) *The Courtament Commitment, Phase 2: First year progress report*, (www.wrap.org.uk/downloads/CC2_First_Year_Progress_Report_05_Dec_11_final.d7cfce64.115474/1).

TWELVE

Conclusions: framing the organising of waste in the city

C. Michael Hall and María José Zapata Campos

Introduction

This concluding chapter now returns to the goal of the book to frame the following synthesis of the main findings from across all the chapters, noting the similarities and dissimilarities between cities, societies and cultures confronted in the book. We conclude with an exploration of the implications drawn for future waste policy governance.

The aim of the book was to emphasise the ways in which the notion of waste, and the narratives and discourses associated with it, are socially constructed with corresponding implications for the governance of waste and the local wasting practices in cities. Below are some tentative responses to this aim in the form of four sets of critical findings.

Global narratives of waste translated into local practices

This book has shown that despite the existence of powerful global narratives of waste, their local translation into household solid waste governance and wasting practices varies over space and time. The existing governmental and institutional arrangements in which the household solid waste governance and practices are embedded play a fundamental role in the local translation of global ideas of waste, as shown in the analysis of waste policies in New Zealand and Ireland (see Chapters Four and Ten). Different waste narratives are also often translated from one jurisdiction to another as part of the processes of policy learning and transfer. Waste governance and waste narratives are part of broader meta-narratives (Lyotard, 1979) such as ideas of consumption, sustainable development, resource scarcity, good governance and competitiveness, all of which might even be more influential in shaping waste management practice than global waste narratives, given that waste policies are often embedded in broad institutional and policy contexts (see Chapter Four). Furthermore, despite waste narratives being relevant, the techno-institutional order in which waste governance occurs also matters. In Ireland, waste governance has to be framed in the context of a society in a rapid transit from an agrarian into an urbanised modern economy, where industrialisation and the production of waste went hand-in-hand. In Cairo, the Zabaleen's waste collectors narrative is an unfinished story (see Chapter Nine). It is framed in a context of radical policy action and contemporary major political events that might change the techno-institutional, as well as more directly the political, order in Egypt in which waste governance is embedded. Again in Ireland (Chapter Four), Anna Davies illustrates how government still matters, and how the structure of public administration and other institutional arrangements make a difference in how waste narratives are locally interpreted.

Finally, the existence of competing narratives both at a societal and at a local level also affect how new and emergent ideas of waste and sociomateriality are locally translated. Liam Leonard and Anna Davies show that the way societies understand and relate to nature (for example, perceiving waste as a natural resource to exploit or as a natural resource to protect and to use in harmony with the environment) remains at the background of environmental policies and regulations and helps explain how certain global narratives of waste prevention might anchor more firmly in some societies than in others. Similarly, C. Michael Hall in Chapter Two highlighted how the perception of land as waste has led to the lack of appreciation of its ecological values. At the local level, the book has shown how the lack of understanding of local narratives and practices of waste, for instance, in informal settlements and less well-off neighbourhoods, leads to counter-productive practices such as residents lighting fires or dumping waste illegally.

This book also evidences how different narratives of waste coexist. The cases explored in this volume have identified a polyphony of voices or narratives regarding what waste is, how it is produced, how we relate to waste and how to govern it. For instance, narratives of zero waste coexist with the Integrated Solid Waste Management (ISWM) and the European hierarchy model. Waste is understood at once as a commodity, as an environmental and health problem, as a critical urban service, or as something that simply should not become. Some of the policy documents analysed in this book put together different and sometimes contradictory narratives of waste. However, contradictory narratives can be very 'effective' in policy terms (Corvellec and Hultman, 2012) given that they have the capability to satisfy different audiences, functions and interests. In this polyphony some voices are heard louder than others. There are some narratives that become dominant, such as traditional ecological modernisation, underscoring the predominant idea that environmental problems, whether waste or global environmental change, are framed by institutions primarily in technical and economic terms rather than as social and/or political problems (Demerrit, 2001, 2006; Scott et al, 2012). This predominant narrative is also reflected in the contradictions faced by the hybrid waste management companies studied in the book, and how profitability is put ahead of the environment. Indeed, the marketisation of waste and the accompanying generation of profits as well as employment opportunities may present a long-term challenge to sustainable consumption. As Patrik Zapata pointed out in Chapter Five, waste policy documents in Managua that framed waste as a resource and not as an environmental problem potentially bring forth the idea that low waste production is bad (as an indicator of underdevelopment), and if a future income of the poor is waste, more and not less waste is needed – which is quite the opposite position from waste prevention.

In EU countries the European waste hierarchy model prioritises waste reduction over reuse and recycle practices. Although rhetorically at least, the waste hierarchy model has been adopted and officially translated into national laws, targets and plans (Chapter Four), the discursive harmony in these all-embracing waste narratives may actually be quite fractured as a result of different national and local interpretations. For example, in many Swedish cities, as well as in many other north European cities, waste incinerators have become the dominant waste infrastructure to handle waste, and are intimately interlocked with municipal district infrastructures created in the post-Second World War period. By contrast, in Ireland waste incineration has not succeeded in becoming significant waste infrastructure, despite the ongoing efforts of the national government, and instead, landfilling continues well beyond the EU permitted targets. In other words, although waste reduction has become a central goal and the emergent narrative in European countries, 'its meaning is more open ended' (Bulkeley and Gregson, 2009: 929). The waste prevention narrative is, as Corvellec and Hultman show in Chapter Eight, not yet as systematically developed in practice, and remains still more a matter of ambitions than of practical solutions.

There are also narratives that do not travel so well, such was the case of zero waste and the limited support collected in the cases presented in this book, which may have substantial implications for global sustainability strategies. Some ideas anchor in local societies better than others, following the reasons discussed above. The development of institutional arrangements, such as meta-organisations (organisations whose members are other organisations) and new forms of multilayered environmental governance, have played a fundamental role in the travel of new narratives of waste through directives, legislation and plans, which are then finally disembedded in such activities as regional waste plans, the construction of infrastructures and the imposition of levies, targets and charges. Mediators such as consultants, non-governmental organisations (NGOs) and experts, as well as non-human mediators such as the texts analysed in this book, or the waste trucks shadowed by Dario Minervini in his home town, make the connection between global narratives and local institutions and practices by connecting interests and meanings. The role of mediators becomes crucial for the good functioning of waste governance and the implementation of policies into practice (Minervini, 2010). There is, however, a dark side of intermediation in waste governance and infrastructures (Marvin et al, 2011). The standardisation of waste governance solutions, such as the elaboration of similar waste regional plans by the participation of the same consultants in Ireland, can result in ignoring local institutional arrangements, interests, values and practices. Furthermore, the particular interests held by these intermediators, such as the case of these consultants, biases the translation of narratives and national waste directives in the detriment of some interests and in favour of others, including their own.

Although the final translations might result in different practices, paths of convergence have also been identified in the book. Financial instruments such as landfill levies, waste regional plans, the creation of national waste packaging producer responsibility initiatives, the construction of similar waste infrastructures such as waste transference stations in Nicaragua or waste incinerators in Europe, were similar solutions adopted in different parts of the world. Differently expressed, the glocalisation of waste narratives has resulted both in allomorphism and isomorphism processes.

Waste narratives and infrastructures for more sustainable urban transformations

Different chapters in this book have also indicated the stubborn linkage between economic growth and waste production. Significantly, it has been noted that this relationship is not just an issue with respect to economic paradigms, but is also related to institutional arrangements. In Chapter Five Patrik Zapata showed how waste was black-boxed (Latour, 1987) in waste policy documents, by focusing only on the collection, transportation and disposal side of the waste management: the production of waste was disconnected from its governance. Similarly, María José Zapata Campos discussed in Chapter Three how efficient waste infrastructures that make waste disappear could paradoxically contribute to hide the steady growth of waste, and the consequences of the 'consume and discard' society.

One of the challenges for achieving more sustainable urban transformations is the decoupling of economic growth from waste production (Mazzanti, 2008; Sjöström and Östblom, 2010; Mazzanti and Nicolli, 2011; D'Amato et al, 2012; Mazzanti et al, 2012; Nicolli et al, 2012). New narratives of waste reduction as well as a number of social practices and environmental policies can operate to re-establish the cognitive links between production, design, consumption and waste, breaking new roads towards a 'wasting less' governance (Corvellec and Hultman, 2012). Making visible the hidden work of waste infrastructures, waste management companies, official waste operators, informal waste pickers and even ordinary citizens is crucial to this end. Recycling containers, school visits or environmental campaigns are practices that may help unlock these hidden infrastructures and services by visualising materially or symbolically the impacts of our consumption practices.

Transition from a 'wasting less' narrative to 'wasting less' practices

The Western societies studied in this book have experienced a transition from a 'less landfilling' towards 'wasting less' waste governance (Chapter Eight). Yet waste prevention policies are not as developed in practice (Mazzanti and Nicolli, 2011). Rather, they are still more a goal and an ambition, present at a discourse level, than a solution. As Mazzanti and Nicolli (2011: 61) note in the case of the EU, 'although absolute decoupling is far from being generally achieved for both municipal and even packaging waste generation … there are some first positive signs of stronger relative decoupling with respect to the past. Nevertheless, the impact of waste policies is negligible, probably due to the biased focus on waste disposal and recovery rather than waste reduction at source.'

Notwithstanding the limited rate of change, it is clear that the waste prevention and reduction narratives are challenging the established waste governance order (Corvellec and Hultman, 2012). The environmental policies and social practices mentioned above also indicate changes in the sociomaterial modes of how we understand waste and how we relate to it (Gregson, 2009; Corvellec and Hultman, 2012; Hultman and Corvellec, 2012). Furthermore, the EU waste hierarchy and the derived European and national directives will continue to enact a significant influence on the shape of waste management practices in European countries,gradually bringing waste prevention to the top of this hierachy.

It is in transitions like this journey towards 'wasting less' modes of governance, when openings for the introduction of new values, ideas, narratives or infrastructures emerge. Challengers such as civil society organisations, environmental movements, researchers or waste collectors associations can introduce their values, interests and practices. Technological, institutional and social forces co-produce a techno-institutional complex that prevents the diffusion of more sustainable technologies, infrastructures and modes of governance to transform and reduce waste at source. This 'lock-in' (Unruh, 2000) can, however, be unlocked. And even cultural and cognitive changes, such as the introduction of new waste reduction narratives, have an unlocking potential (Corvellec et al, 2012). New views on waste challenge the existing dominant societal narrative that waste is a valuable resource to be exploited, and suggest instead that waste is something that should not be produced (Bulkeley and Gregson, 2009; Corvellec et al, 2012). New ways to relate to waste are being developed in households, in civil society organisations or from scholars visiting waste infrastructures. These new forms of sociomateriality offer civil society organisations, environmental parties and movements, but also waste management companies, opportunities for unlocking sociotechnical innovations. The environmental challenge is to move towards 'wasting less' governance regimes by reconnecting and bridging (materially and symbolically) production, consumption and waste production. For example, in Managua and Cairo, the sociomaterial achievement was the commodification of waste, the assignment of legitimate economic value, which was also extended to those informally collecting and transforming waste. Making waste collection, material and energy recovery more efficient remain the main goals in the Nicaraguan case, especially in a city like Managua, where a functioning waste management system has to be secured in order to preserve public health and to support the economic activities in the city. However, Zapata (Chapter Five) observed that waste reduction was absent in the studied policy documents, missing the opportunity to use the visible sociomateriality of waste to promote waste prevention in a manner that not only promoted sustainable consumption but also provided transition paths for those who currently depend on waste commodification.

Waste narratives, infrastructures, governance and power

In the potential transition to waste reduction it seems that in the contemporary political-economic environment waste governance will be increasingly linked to the business-oriented agenda of efficiency and competitiveness. Consequently, trends towards economic instruments and privatisation of waste management through hybrid waste management companies, and the emergence of multinational corporations operating as local waste operators, will probably increase, especially when driving forces are more than ever efficiency and fiscal austerity (see Chapter Four). As a consequence, public control over the environmental management of waste through hybrid and private organisations, the conflict between economic and environmental values and the difficulties of governing a highly technological infrastructure that demands increasing levels of specialised knowledge will remain as central issues of waste governance in the foreseeable future.

Another aspect of power brought up in several chapters in this book is how waste management companies work on getting people to subject themselves to the discourse and practical order of governmentality (Foucault, 1991; Dean, 1999) that companies design, with clear sets of categories, classification, priorities, moral obligations, rewards and penalties (Chapter Eight). This is how, at the micro level, waste management companies exhort householders to look at their waste: to recognise it, name it, classify it and separate it. They do this by designing the sociomateriality of waste, through pricing, marketing, recycling practices and so on. Among other things, waste management companies teach us how to make our own waste both visible and invisible.

Corvellec and Hultman (2012: 302) ask: 'for whom is this (waste) a problem, and for whom is it a resource?' In this book it has been shown how waste is generally a problem for all, considering issues of resource scarcity, pollution and climate change, but it is a more concrete problem for some people and some places. Waste is a problem for the waste pickers or the waste collectors undertaking their work in poor working conditions, for the residents living close to a landfill site or a waste incinerator, or for the city dwellers of informal settlements and less well-off areas with worse, inexistent or inadequate waste collection services. Waste is also a resource 'for those who solve the waste problem' (Corvellec and Hultman, 2012: 302). In the redistribution of the benefits of the commoditisation of waste, multinational corporations often unfairly compete with informal waste collectors as a result of waste privatisation policies. In this book the interests of the waste packing industry in not reducing but increasing waste packing production has also been discussed. Waste prevention is in the discourse of national waste policies. However, in practice, waste packaging is also increasing as a business and as a cost to citizens, and especially of citizens of less well-off areas. The power struggle regarding packaging waste remains an example of the challenges for the multilevel governance of complex waste interests. Increasing the recycling rates in households remains a meaningless solution if the amount of waste packaging, and the economic interests behind it, do not stop growing. At a regional and a global level, the uneven geographies of waste in time and space also raise issues of environmental injustice (Davies, 2008), with respect to the mobility of waste beyond national frontiers, between fluctuating markets and to stages in the flow of waste where waste is shipped to directly because of poor environmental regulation and employment conditions, and hence, low costs of 'disposal'.

Future policy implications

Although paths of policy convergence, standardisation, imitation and compliance have been identified in this volume, ordinary householders, informal waste collectors or environmental civil society organisations have also contested waste policies and governance. National waste policies, laws, plans and programmes have to acknowledge local waste practices, including illegal and informal waste practices, the coexistence of different modes of sociomateriality and the social, economic and cultural differences that exist, even within cities. This understanding becomes crucial in the translation of supranational, national and regional environmental directives related to the governance of waste to local interests and practices. This implies a more comprehensive, yet open and flexible waste governance regime that supports the translation of global ideas of waste into different national and local contexts (Nicolli et al, 2012).

The increasing role of hybrid waste management companies and waste multinational corporations demands further control and scrutiny from the public sector to guarantee that profitability does not diminish the likelihood of achieving environmental and social goals, including securing greater levels of environmental justice in cities. Similarly, waste governance regimes that seek to implement waste reduction approaches require better control over the mediators that support the connections between the actors involved in the processes of production, consumption, waste collection and handling. Furthermore, waste governance needs to leverage the conditions where mediators can enact practical, flexible and innovative solutions through positive intermediation, so as to prevent processes of 'lock-in' whereby sustainable innovations are excluded for waste management regimes and systems (Marvin et al, 2011).

In order to be effective, urban waste policies and plans have to understand how informal waste collection practices are entrenched within formal collection services and multinational corporations. This means that waste governance has to acknowledge the sociomaterialities of waste, meaning how individuals relate to waste, and therefore design waste categories, priorities, moral obligations, rewards and penalties so as to encourage positive individual behaviour towards more sustainable urban and societal transformations (Barr, 2008). Current research related to how individuals relate to consumption and disposal within and outside our households (see, for example, Bulkeley and Gregson, 2009; Hall, 2011; Lane and Gorman-Murray, 2011) can shed light on more sustainable modes of local waste governance. Furthermore, waste laws and policies have to operate towards a fair redistribution, both of costs and benefits of waste policies. This especially includes tackling the core of the waste problem, which is the growth of the amount of waste. As noted above, the reduction of waste packaging and food waste are important targets in European and other waste policies, which have the challenge of being translated into practice (Coggins, 2001; Mazzanti and Nicolli, 2011; Tasaki and Yamakawa, 2011; Hall and Gössling, 2013).

Waste reduction or 'wasting less' is the emergent societal narrative that although primarily attached to Europe is of enormous global significance given its role in sustainable consumption and degrowth. Although at the time of writing it is at more of a discursive level than in practice, it is expected that waste reduction will become more and more part of local and national waste practices. The societal narratives, ideas and values to make waste unbecome are already here. Within Europe the regulations to translate this narrative are also approved in EU and national directives translating the European waste hierarchy. However, to lock out the predominant techno-institutional order towards more sustainable urban transformations it is also necessary to change the economic conditions (with the associated economic interests), to develop more efficient and locally contextualised policy instruments and to change the physical infrastructure that makes them possible (which are often the most expensive and slow to change; see Corvellec et al, 2012). Nevertheless, local institutions, city authorities and waste management companies will need to get ready for this transition towards new modes of waste governance where reduction becomes central for local practice.

The increasing role of supranational and national environmental regulations have arguably reduced the decision and policy-making space of local governments, which has evolved towards the regionalisation of the environmental management of issues, such as waste (Davoudi and Evans, 2005). City authorities face a new techno-institutional order in which they have to redefine their roles. In this process of adjustment, in countries like Sweden municipalities increasingly demand the devolution of, for example, the collection of waste packaging, arguing that public authorities will defend more effectively and fairly the principle of waste minimisation over the profit made by the waste recycling industry. The reconsideration of the widespread solution of putting the private sector in the driving seat of such a task could also play a central role in the challenge of minimising the growing mountain of waste that contributes to global environmental change.

Finally, although touched on at times in this book, one of the most pressing needs is to understand waste within the broader context of consumption and production. However, as has been stressed throughout, waste reduction and prevention is part of the broader circulation and flow of materials around the planet and their use and exchange values. To promote waste prevention is to challenge not only the dominant ways of thinking about packaging and physical products, but is actually a direct challenge to business as usual – full stop – given that it affects how we produce and consume things and how far products or consumers have to travel for the consumptive act to be consummated.

In thinking about the sociomateriality of waste and the various narratives of waste, we are therefore encouraging such approaches as a valuable means to cast a wider lens on the problem of sustainability. As has been stressed throughout, technical-rational economic and engineering approaches have not been successful in dealing with waste; in fact, the marketisation of waste has only created its own set of problems and has perhaps made waste prevention even more difficult than it already is. Instead, social sciences research has great capacity to better understand why technical 'solutions' play out the way they do and help find ways to make them better fit varying local circumstances without undesired externalities or opportunity costs. In exactly the same way, the problem of sustainable development and consumption cannot be 'solved' by neoclassical economics and engineering. Technical innovations and greater efficiencies are extremely important, but they need to be matched by an understanding of sufficiency and the slowing of rates of material circulation. These are areas where the critical social sciences approach can be of great value in ensuring that the construction of new regimes of sustainability, and hence the global and local material flows of waste through the city, are grounded not just in technical innovations but also social innovations that value economic, environmental and social justice.

References

Barr, S. (2008) *Environment and society: Sustainability, policy and the citizen*, Aldershot: Ashgate.

Bulkeley, H. and Gregson, N. (2009) 'Crossing the threshold: municipal waste policy and household waste generation', *Environment and Planning A*, vol 41, pp 929-45.

Coggins, C. (2001) 'Waste prevention – an issue of shared responsibility for UK producers and consumers: policy options and measurement', *Resources, Conservation and Recycling*, vol 32, nos 3-4, pp 181-90.

Corvellec, H. and Hultman, J. (2012) 'From "less landfilling" to "wasting less": Societal narratives, socio-materiality, and organizations', *Journal of Organizational Change Management*, vol 25, no 2, pp 297-314.

Corvellec, H., Zapata Campos, M.J. and Zapata, P. (2012) 'Infrastructures, lock-in, and sustainable urban development – the case of waste incineration in a Swedish metropolitan area', *Journal of Cleaner Production*, http://dx.doi.org/10.1016/j.jclepro.2012.12.009

D'Amato, A., Managi, S. and Mazzanti, M. (2012) 'Economics of waste management and disposal: decoupling, policy enforcement and spatial factors', *Environmental Economics and Policy Studies*, vol 14, pp 323-5.

Davies, A. (2008) *Geographies of garbage governance: Interventions, interactions and outcomes*, Aldershot: Ashgate.

Davoudi, S. and Evans, N. (2005) 'The challenge of governance in regional waste planning', *Environment and Planning C: Government and Policy*, vol 23, no 4, pp 493-519.

Dean, M. (1999) *Governmentality: Power and rule in modern society*, Thousand Oaks, CA: Sage.

Demeritt, D. (2001) 'The construction of global warming and the politics of science', *Annals of the Association of American Geographers*, vol 91, pp 307-37.

Demeritt, D. (2006) 'Science studies, climate change and the prospects for constructivist critique', *Economy and Society*, vol 35, pp 453-79.

Foucault, M. (1991) 'Governmentality', trans. Rosi Braidotti and revised by Colin Gordon, in G. Burchell, C. Gordon and P. Miller (eds) *The Foucault effect: Studies in governmentality*, pp 87–104. Chicago, IL: University of Chicago Press.

Gössling, S. and Hall, C.M. (2013) 'Sustainable culinary systems: An introduction', in S. Gössling, S. and C.M. Hall, C.M. (eds) *Sustainable culinary systems: Local foods, innovation, and tourism and hospitality*, London: Routledge, pp 3-44.

Gregson, N. (2009) 'Recycling as policy and assemblage', *Geography*, vol 94, no 1, pp 61-5.

Hall, C.M. (2011) 'Consumerism, tourism and voluntary simplicity: We all have to consume, but do we really have to travel so much to be happy?', *Tourism Recreation Research*, vol 36, no 3, 298-303.

Hall, C.M. (2013) 'The natural science ontology of environment', in A. Holden and D. Fennell (eds) *The Routledge handbook of tourism and the environment*, London: Routledge.

Hultman, J. and Corvellec, H. (2012) 'The waste hierarchy model: from the socio-materiality of waste to a politics of consumption', *Environment and Planning A*, vol 44, no 10, pp 2413-27.

Lane, R. and Gorman-Murray, A. (eds) (2011) *Material geographies of the household*, Aldershot: Ashgate.

Latour, B. (1987) *Science in action: How to follow scientists and engineers through society*, Milton Keynes: Open University Press.

Lyotard, J.-F. (1979) *The postmodern condition: A report on knowledge*, Manchester: Manchester University Press.

Marvin, S., Guy, S., Medd, W. and Moss, T. (2011) 'Conclusions: The transformative power of intermediaries', in S. Guy, S. Marvin, W. Medd and T. Moss (eds) *Shaping urban infrastructures: Intermediaries and the governance of socio-technical networks*, London: Earthscan.

Mazzanti, M. (2008) 'Is waste generation de-linking from economic growth? Empirical evidence for Europe', *Applied Economics Letters*, vol 15, no 4, pp 287-91.

Mazzanti, M. and Nicolli, F. (2011) 'Waste dynamics, decoupling and ex-post policy effectiveness: Evidence from the EU15', *International Journal of Global Environmental Issues*, vol 11, no 1, pp 61-78.

Mazzanti, M., Montini, A. and Nicolli, F. (2012) 'Waste dynamics in economic and policy transitions: decoupling, convergence and spatial effects', *Journal of Environmental Planning and Management*, vol 55, no 5, pp 563-81.

Minervini, D. (2010) *Politica e rifiuti. Connessioni socio-tecniche nella governance dell'ambiente*, Napoli: Linguori Editore.

Nicolli , F., Mazzanti, M. and Iafolla, V. (2012) 'Waste dynamics, country heterogeneity and European environmental policy effectiveness', *Journal of Environmental Policy & Planning*, vol 14, no 4, 371-93.

Scott, D., Gössling, S. and Hall, C.M. (2012) *Tourism and climate change: Impacts, adaptation and mitigation*, London: Routledge.

Sjöström, M. and Östblom, G. (2010) 'Decoupling waste generation from economic growth – A CGE analysis of the Swedish case', *Ecological Economics*, vol 69, no 7, pp 1545-52.

Tasaki, T. and Yamakawa, H. (2011) 'An estimation of the effectiveness of waste prevention by using point-of-sales (POS) data – The case of refills for shampoo and hair conditioner in Japan', *Resources, Conservation and Recycling*, vol 57, pp 61-6.

Unruh, C. (2000) 'Understanding carbon lock-in', *Energy Policy*, vol 28, no 12, pp 817-30.

Index

D

E

J

L

M

N